THE RUNNING ATHLETE: ROENTGENOGRAMS AND REMEDIES

The Running Athlete: Roentgenograms and Remedies

HELENE PAVLOV, M.D.
Attending Radiologist
Department of Radiology and Nuclear Medicine
Hospital for Special Surgery
Associate Professor of Radiology
Cornell University Medical College
Associate Attending Radiologist
New York Hospital
New York, New York

JOSEPH S. TORG, M.D.
Professor of Orthopaedic Surgery
Director, Sports Medicine Center
University of Pennsylvania School of Medicine
Philadelphia, Pennsylvania

YEAR BOOK MEDICAL PUBLISHERS, INC.
Chicago • London • Boca Raton

1 2 3 4 5 6 7 8 9 0 CK 91 90 89 88 87

Library of Congress Cataloging-in-Publication Data

Pavlov, Helene.
　The running athlete.

　Includes bibliographies and index.
　1. Extremities, Lower—Wounds and injuries—
Diagnosis.　2. Spine—Wounds and injuries—Diagnosis.
3. Diagnosis, Radioscopic.　4. Extremities, Lower—
Wounds and injuries—Treatment.　5. Spine—Wounds and
injuries—Treatment.　6. Running—Accidents and
injuries.　I. Torg, Joseph S.　II. Title.　[DNLM:
1. Athletic Injuries—radiography—atlases.
2. Athletic Injuries—therapy—atlases.　3. Running—
atlases.　QT 17 P338r]
RD560.P38　1986　　　617′.1027　　　86-15943
ISBN 0-8151-6712-1

Sponsoring Editor: James D. Ryan, Jr.

Manager, Copyediting Services: Frances M. Perveiler

Production Project Manager: Max Perez

Proofroom Supervisor: Shirley E. Taylor

To the very best part of my life, Harvey Zeichner, Esq.—H.P.

and

My gang, Barbara, Joe Jr., Betsy, Jay, Hercules and Dusty.—J.S.T.

Foreword

"Well, in our country," said Alice, still panting a little, "you'd generally get to somewhere else—if you ran very fast for a long time as we've been doing."

"A slow sort of country!" said the Queen. "Now, here, you see, it takes all the running you can do, to keep in the same place. If you want to get somewhere else, you must run at least twice as fast as that!"

Through the Looking Glass, Lewis Carroll

Running to catch animals for food and to escape from being the food of larger animals—once a principal activity of humans—has been replaced by other, faster forms of locomotion, and running to carry messages beyond the range of the voice is no longer necessary. But the death of the runner who carried the victory message from Marathon to Athens has not been forgotten, and is a reminder that running for sport or pleasure is not without its medical complications.

Today running is part of every athletic endeavor and is by itself a simple and relatively inexpensive sport that keeps the locomotor and cardiovascular systems, as well as the mental state of the runner, in good order. "Mens sana in corporo sano," means "a healthy mind in a healthy body," as the old Romans used to say. Perhaps because running is exhilarating and produces the pleasurable "runners high," amateurs may run faster and farther than their training and physical condition allow, but the physical complications of running are by no means confined to the poorly trained, overage or overweight amateur. Professional athletes in competition perform at levels that overtax the well-conditioned musculoskeletal system. Stress injuries in players of basketball, a game that demands an incredible amount of running and jumping, have become the rule rather than the exception. These otherwise minor injuries are devastating to both performance and income of professional athletes. As the authors point out, many sports-related injuries are difficult to diagnose in their early stages when they are treatable by nonsurgical means. Early diagnosis and treatment can prevent the prolonged or permanent disability that cuts short the career of the professional athlete and can severely limit the activity of amateur athletes.

ROBERT H. FREIBERGER, M.D.

Preface

This book is dedicated and devoted to the trials and tribulations of the running athlete. As this person stands before us with a full head of unkempt hair, shopping bag full of malodorous running shoes in one arm, and in the other, an exquisitely compulsive documented chronology of every "injury," twinge of pain, and discomfort, real and imagined, that has been suffered over the past 18 months, we, the athlete's physicians, more times than not remain totally befuddled by his complaints, demands, and pleas for sympathy and compassion at the height of our harried and busy day. To deal with this problem is an exercise in frustration, many times completely draining both our physical and intellectual resources. The athlete has run 120 miles this week and is attempting to prepare for the upcoming marathon, but for unidentified reasons is hampered by "injury" that, although acute and well localized, defies diagnosis and subsequent treatment. Logic would tell us that rest is the answer; however, the patient refuses to stop his inordinate exercise and physical self-abuse.

Physical examination reveals that the athlete's feet are flat, knees are knocked, excessive femoral anteversion is present, and to top it off, one lower extremity is 3mm longer than its mate. What can we do? What can we do to enable our "athlete" to discontinue this masochistic course of self-inflicted physical abuse and mental anguish?

In keeping with basic principles of good medical practice, a diagnosis is always helpful. It is to this end that this volume, *The Running Athlete: Roentgenograms and Remedies*, is devoted. Hopefully, with the implementation of proper roentgenographic and other imaging techniques, the physician will be better able to identify the underlying problem so as to initiate implementation of appropriate therapeutic measures.

JOSEPH S. TORG, M.D.

Contents

CHAPTER 1
The Foot

UNGUAL TUFT

Subungual Exostosis

Subungual exostosis are large, bony projections from the dorsal surface of the ungual tuft.

FIG 1–1.
A, B, Two examples. The size and shape of these projections vary. (Permission for **A, B** granted courtesy of Pavlov H, Torg JS, Hersh A, et al: The roentgen examination of runners' injuries. *RadioGraphics* 1981; 1:17–34.)

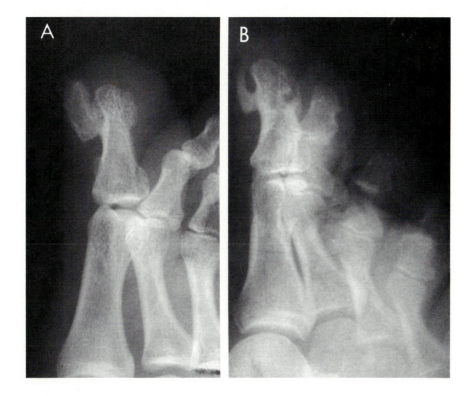

Subungual Exostosis

REMEDY   Padding and shoe modification, trim nail back, and/or excision of exostosis.

SESAMOIDS

Normal Variation

The individual fragments of bipartite and multipartite sesamoids have corticated, beveled margins and the fragments do not "fit" together.

FIG 1–2.
A, Variations of sesamoids in descending order of frequency. (Permission for **A** granted courtesy of Feldman P, Pochaczevsky P, Hecht H: The case of the wandering sesamoid and other sesamoid afflictions. *Radiology* 1970; 96:275–283.)

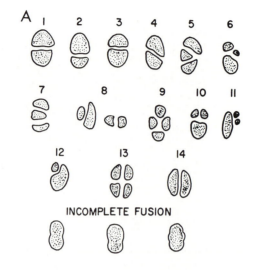

INCOMPLETE FUSION

B, Bilateral bipartite medial sesamoids.
C, Typical bipartite medial and fibular sesamoids. *(Continued.)*

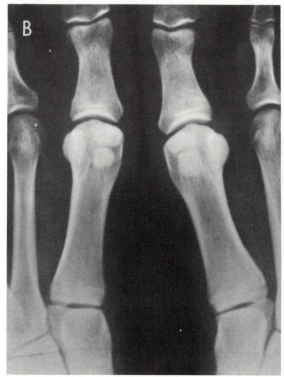

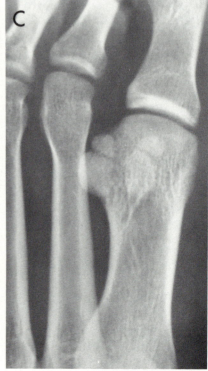

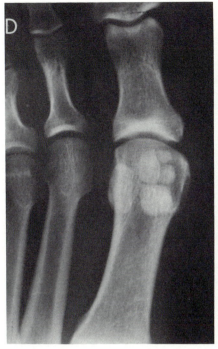

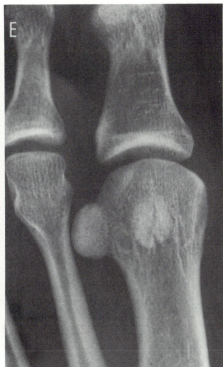

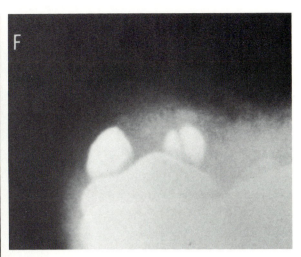

FIG 1–2 (cont.).
D, A multipartite medial sesamoid.
E, A vertical bipartite medial sesamoid.
F, A vertical bipartite fibular sesamoid on an axial view.

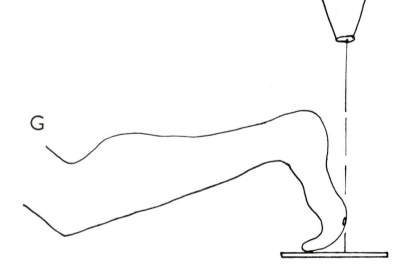

G, The axial view is performed with the central ray tangent to the sesamoid metatarsal joint.

Normal Sesamoid Variation

REMEDY   None, unless symptomatic. Chondromalacia of the sesamoids is not demonstrable on radiographs and has a negative bone scan. *Symptomatic chondromalacia* is treated with a felt "donut" pad, proper shoeing, and decreased activity.

Sesamoid Fracture

FIG 1–3.
A, A horizontal fracture in the fibular sesamoid simulates a bipartite sesamoid except that the fragments "fit" together and the margins along the radiolucency are sharp, not beveled.
B (same patient as **A**), A follow-up examination demonstrates widening of the radiolucent line representing resorption along the fracture margin.

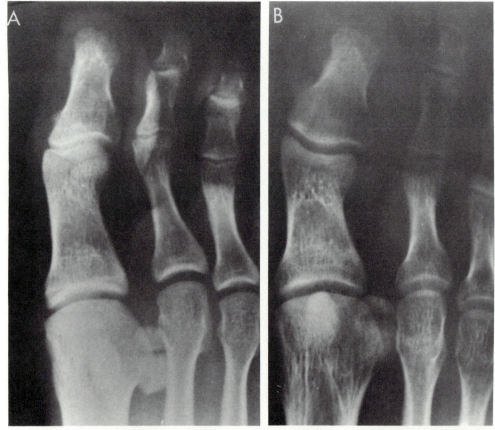

C,D, Two examples of comminuted nondisplaced fractures *(arrows)* of the fibular sesamoid. *(Continued.)*

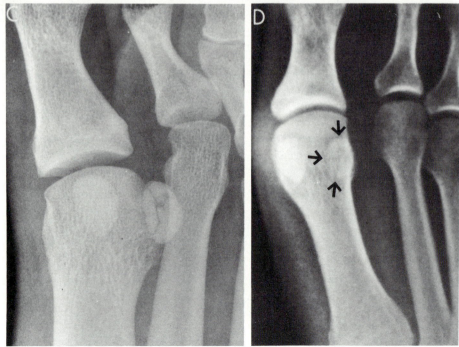

FIG 1–3 (cont.).
E, An axial view demonstrates a nondisplaced fracture of the medial sesamoid *(arrow).*

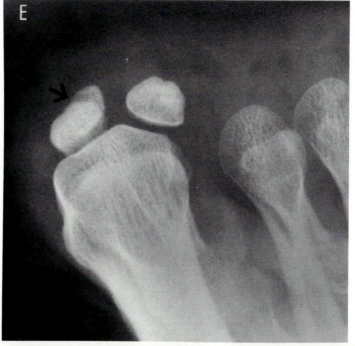

F,G (both same patient), Frontal and axial views demonstrate a slightly displaced horizontal fracture *(arrow)* of the medial sesamoid. *(Continued.)*

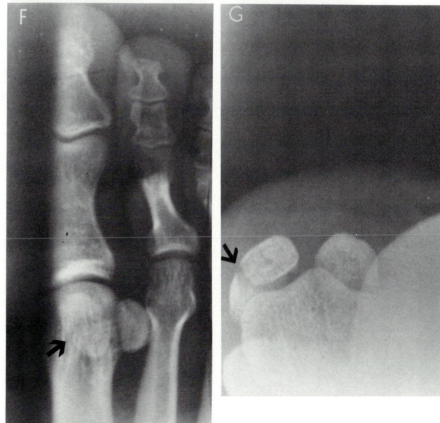

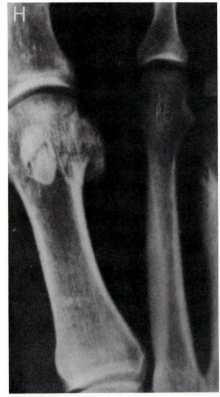

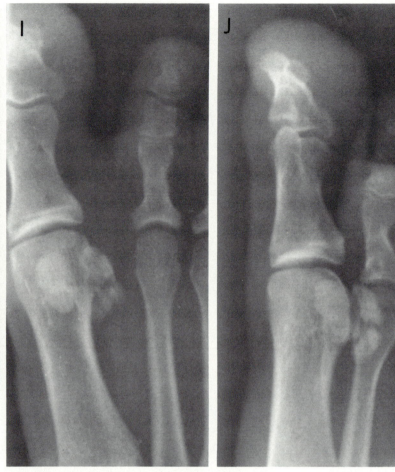

FIG 1–3 (cont.).
H, Horizontal fractures through both the medial and fibular sesamoids.

I,J (both same patient), Frontal and oblique views demonstrate a comminuted crush fracture of the bipartite fibular sesamoid. The medial sesamoid is bipartite.

Sesamoid Fracture

REMEDY

The differentiation of an *acute fracture* from a *stress fracture* of the sesamoid is the patient's history; an acute fracture has a sudden onset of pain compared with a stress fracture that presents with an insidious onset.

Acute fractures of the sesamoid should be treated by non-weight-bearing with crutches for 3 to 6 weeks. In the running athlete, it has been established that *stress fractures* will not heal with conservative management and consideration of excision of the involved sesamoid is recommended. *In instances of nonunion* of either an acute fracture or a stress fracture, with or without degenerative changes, excision of the sesamoid is recommended. (Ref: Van Hal ME, Keene JS, Lange TA, et al: Stress fractures of the great toe sesamoids. *Am J Sports Med* 1982; 10:122.

Distraction of Sesamoid Fragments

Distraction of the sesamoid fragments is diagnosed by an abnormal orientation and/or separation between either bipartite or fracture fragments.

FIG 1–4.
A, Distraction of fibular sesamoid fragments.
B, Distraction of medial sesamoid fragments.

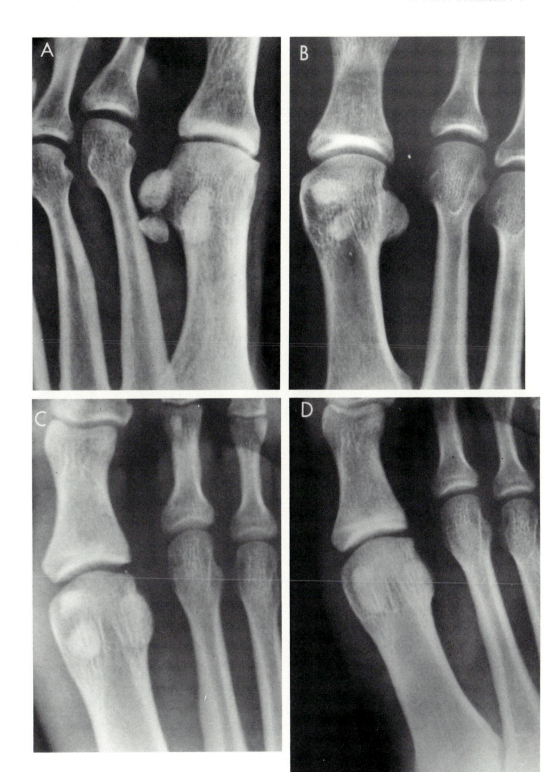

C, D (both same patient), Distraction of medial bipartite fragments, not present on prior films. (Permission for **A–D** granted courtesy of Pavlov H, Torg JS, Hersh A, et al: The roentgen examination of runners' injuries. *RadioGraphics* 1981; 1:17–34.)

FIG 1–4 (cont.).
E, Distraction of the medial sesamoid fragments and a comminuted crush fracture of the proximal portion of the fibular sesamoid.

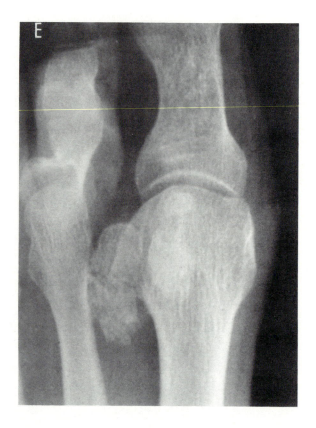

Distraction of Sesamoid Fragments

REMEDY

If symptomatic, treat with a felt "donut" pad, proper shoeing, and decreased activity. If nonresponsive to conservative management, excision of both fragments is recommended.

Sesamoid/Metatarsal Degenerative Osteoarthritis

Osteoarthritic changes occur between the sesamoids and the metatarsal head and consist of joint space narrowing, hypertrophic spurs, and marginal sclerosis.

FIG 1–5.
A,B,C (all same patient), On the AP and oblique views the fibular sesamoid appears enlarged.

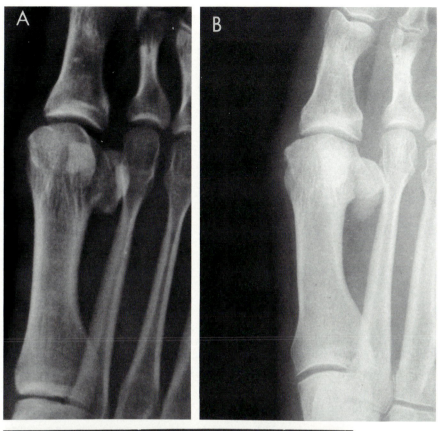

C, On the axial view, all the changes described above of degenerative osteoarthritis are evident between the fibular sesamoid and the metatarsal head. *(Continued.)*

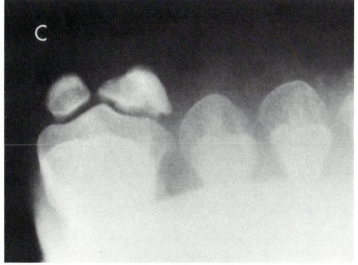

FIG 1–5 (cont.). D,E (both same patient), Frontal and oblique views demonstrate a fragmented fibular sesamoid.

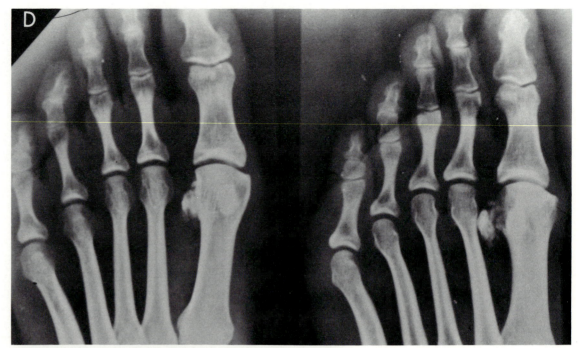

E, An axial view demonstrates fragmentation of the fibular sesamoid with post-traumatic osteoarthritic changes.

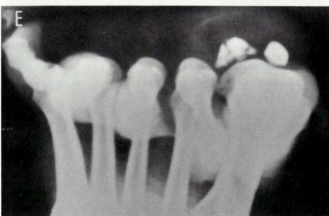

Sesamoid/Metatarsal Degenerative Osteoarthritis

REMEDY   Conservative treatment with a felt "donut" pad, careful shoeing and decreased activity. If symptoms are unresponsive, excision of the sesamoid.

Sesamoid Necrosis

FIG 1–6.
A,B, Two examples: necrosis of the medial sesamoid. The sesamoid is small with an increase in radiodensity and fragmentation. (Ref: Ogata K, Sugioka, Urano Y, et al: Idiopathic osteonecrosis of the first metatarsal sesamoid. *Skeletal Radiol* 1986; 15:141–145.)

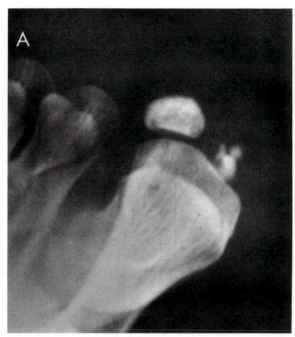 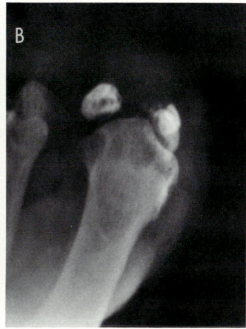

Sesamoid Necrosis

REMEDY   Excise necrotic sesamoid fragments.

Sesamoid Subluxation

FIG 1–7.
A, There is a vertical fracture of the tibial sesamoid. Both fragments are radiodense or "white" compared to the surrounding bones, indicating necrosis.
B (same patient as **A**), On the axial view, the necrotic fragments of the medial sesamoid are distracted. The fibular sesamoid is laterally subluxed with respect to the lateral metatarsal sulcus.

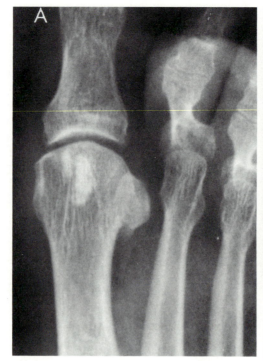

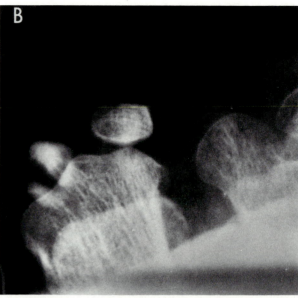

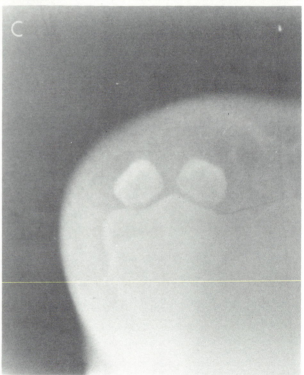

C, Normal alignment of the medial and fibular sesamoids with the metatarsal sulci shown for comparison.

Sesamoid Subluxation

REMEDY   For the subluxed sesamoid, conservative treatment consisting of decreased activity, felt "donut," and careful shoeing; excision may be necessary.

METATARSAL PHALANGEAL JOINT

Bunion

A bunion is a metatarsal adductus primus combined with a hallux valgus. A metatarsal adductus primus indicates an angle greater than 15 degrees between the first metatarsal and the other metatarsals. A hallux valgus is the lateral angulation of the phalange greater than 15 degrees with the longitudinal axis of the metatarsal shaft.

FIG 1–8.
There is a bunion with proliferative hypertrophic spurs and joint space narrowing. (Permission granted courtesy of Pavlov H, Torg JS, Hersh A, et al: The roentgen examination of runners' injuries. *RadioGraphics* 1981; 1:17–34.)

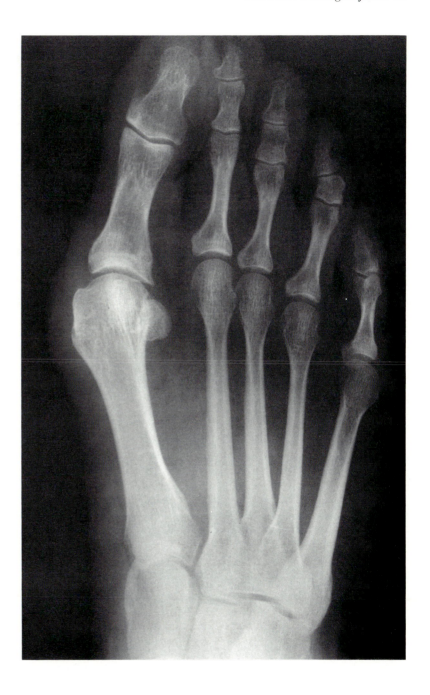

Bunion

REMEDY   Spacers between the first and second toes, padding, steroid injection, and possible simple bunionectomy are appropriate when the intermetatarsal angle is less than 15 degrees. In those patients with an intermetatarsal angle greater than 15 degrees and unresponsive to conservative measurements, the variety and complexity of surgical alternatives are numerous and beyond the scope of this discussion.

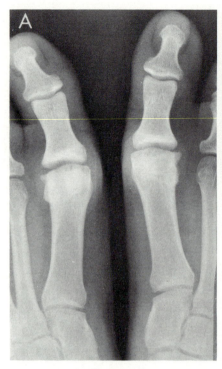

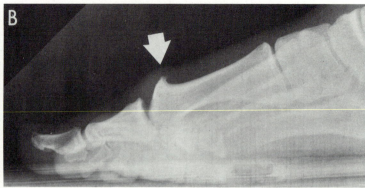

B (same patient as **A**), The dorsal osteophyte (*arrow*) is best seen on the lateral view.

Hallux Rigidus

Hallux rigidus consists of narrowing of the metatarsal phalangeal joints, marginal hypertrophic spurring on the metatarsal heads, and a dorsal osteophyte.

FIG 1–9.
A, Bilateral hallux rigidus.

Hallux Rigidus

REMEDY   Decreased activity, stiff shoe, and possible excision of the dorsal exostosis. *Hallux rigidus* should be differentiated from *hallux limitus.* Hallux limitus is symptomatic decreased motion of the joint due to capsular contracture. The x-rays are normal. Hallux limitus usually responds to range of motion exercises, i.e., metatarsal phalangeal dorsiflexion, and a stiffer shoe.

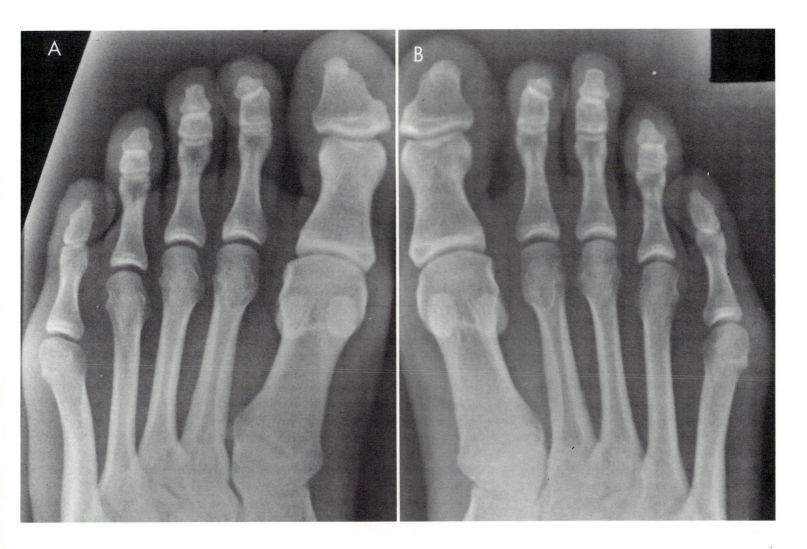

Bunionette

FIG 1–10.
A,B (both same patient), Bilateral bunionette deformities. There is soft tissue swelling lateral to the metatarsal phalangeal joint of the fifth digits. There is slight lateral bowing of the distal aspect of the fifth metatarsals.

Bunionette

REMEDY   Proper shoeing, steroid injection, activity modification, and surgery if patient is unresponsive to conservative management.

METATARSALS

Alignment

Normal Alignment

FIG 1–11.
A, Line connecting the articular surfaces of the metatarsal heads normally forms a gentle arch. The phalanges extend in a straight line from the respective metatarsals and the metatarsals are approximately parallel to each other, extending from a slightly narrow base. (Permission for **A** granted courtesy of Pavlov H, Torg JS, Hersh A, et al: The roentgen examination of runners' injuries. *RadioGraphics* 1981; 1:17–34.) *(Continued.)*

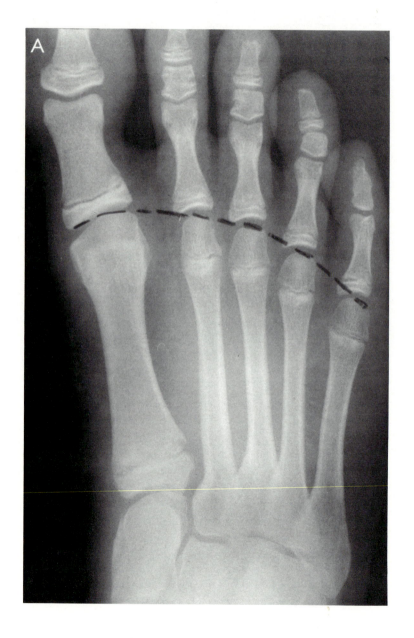

Morton-Type Alignment

FIG 1–11 (cont.).
B, The metatarsal arch is interrupted by a short first metatarsal. The thickening and hyperostosis of the cortex of the second metatarsal shaft, secondary to altered weight bearing stresses, is a common associated finding.

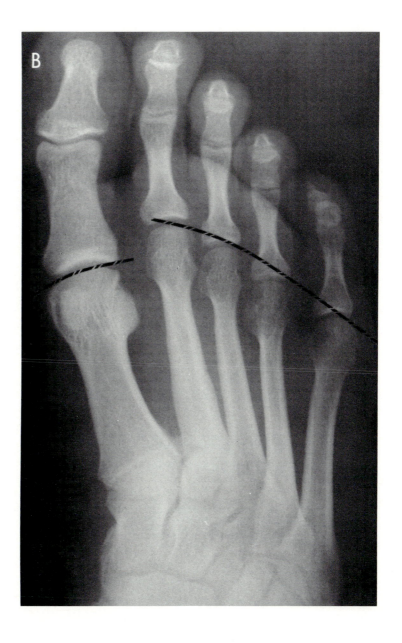

Metatarsal Alignment

REMEDY If a Morton-type foot is symptomatic: decrease activity, reassurance, proper shoes, change in running habits, and orthotics.

Metatarsal Stress Reaction and/or Stress Fracture—Radionuclide Bone Scan

A radionuclide bone scan is a sensitive roentgen modality but it is not specific. It is an excellent means of localizing the site of injury but followup roentgenograms are required to evaluate and appropriately treat the osseous lesion.

FIG 1–12.
A, Localized augmented isotope uptake in the right second metatarsal shaft. (*Continued.*)

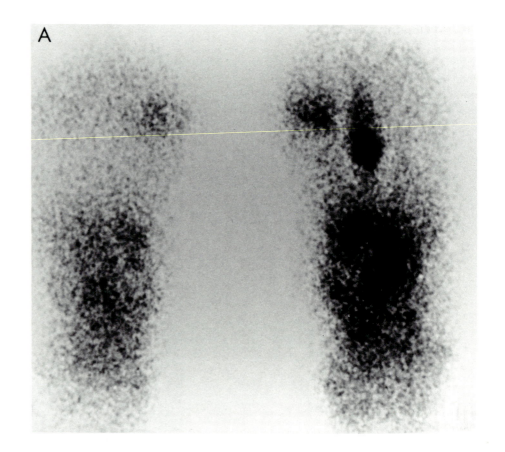

A

FIG 1–12 (cont.).
B, Localized augmented uptake in the second and fourth metatarsal shafts. The uptake in the first metatarsal phalangeal joint corresponds to degenerative changes of the great toe.

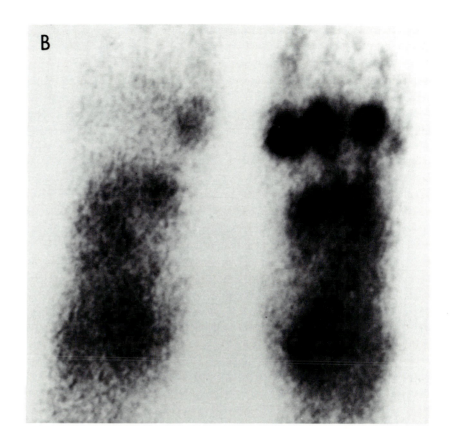

Metatarsal Stress Reaction and/or Stress Fracture

REMEDY Decrease activity, reassurance, proper shoewear, and a change in running habits.

Metatarsal Stress Reaction

A stress reaction is demonstrated radiographically by periosteal new bone formation without a definitive fracture line. Various patterns of periosteal new bone formation and stress reactions of the second metatarsal shaft are demonstrated.

FIG 1–13.
A, Faint periosteal reaction along medial cortex *(arrowheads). (Continued.)*

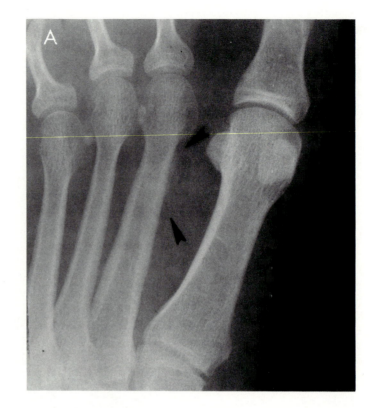

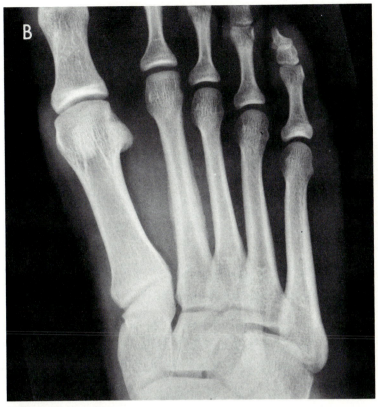

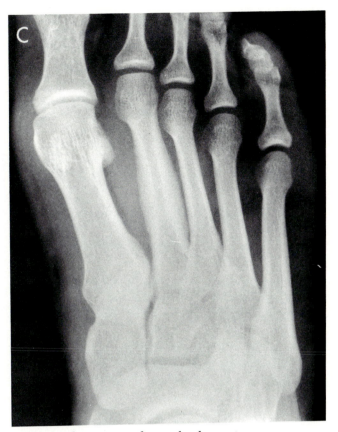

FIG 1–13 (cont.).
B,C (both same patient) Thin layered periosteal new bone formation with endosteal thickening.

C, On a subsequent radiograph, the periosteal and endosteal reaction has matured with marked cortical hypertrophy.

Metatarsal Stress Reaction

REMEDY　　　　　　Decrease activity, reassurance, proper shoes, and a change in running habits.

Metatarsal Stress Fracture—Typical

A stress fracture of the metatarsal is demonstrated radiographically by a radiolucent line within an area of cortical hyperostosis usually involves only one cortex. Various patterns of stress fractures in the second metatarsal are demonstrated.

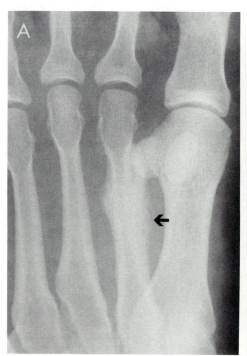 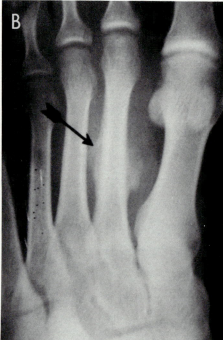 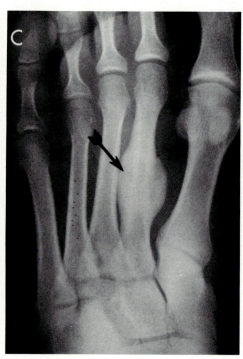

FIG 1–14.

A, A small horizontal radiolucent line *(arrow)* within the medial component of thick fluffy periosteal reaction.

B, An oblique radiolucent fracture *(arrow)* in the lateral component of fluffy periosteal new bone formation.

C, A subsequent radiograph (same patient as **B**) demonstrates maturation of the new bone formation, although the fracture line *(arrow)* within the hyperostosis has not completely healed. *(Continued.)*

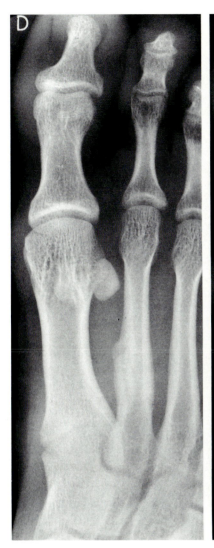
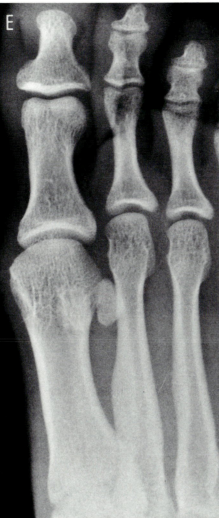
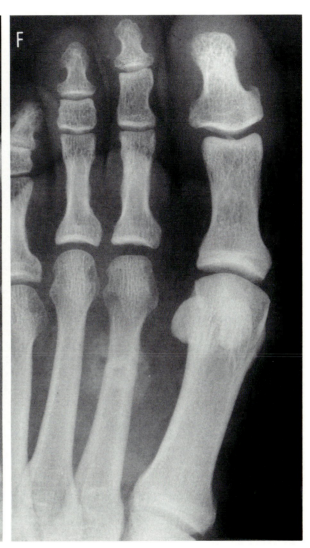

FIG 1–14 (cont.).
D,E (both same patient), Horizontal and vertical radiolucent fractures within the localized area of hyperostosis and thickening of the medial cortex.
E, On a subsequent radiograph the stress fracture has healed with a persistent area of localized cortical thickening.
F, Exuberent callus must be differentiated from periosteal reaction; a fluffy ball of callus around the metatarsal shaft indicates a stress fracture instead of a stress reaction even though the radiolucent line is not visible.

Metatarsal Stress Fracture—Typical

REMEDY   Decrease activity, reassurance, proper shoes, and a change in running habits. Immobilization and non-weight-bearing are generally unnecessary.

Metatarsal Stress Fracture—Complete

Rarely, a stress fracture propagates completely across the bone shaft. The fracture occurs in an area of localized cortical hyperostosis involving both corticles.

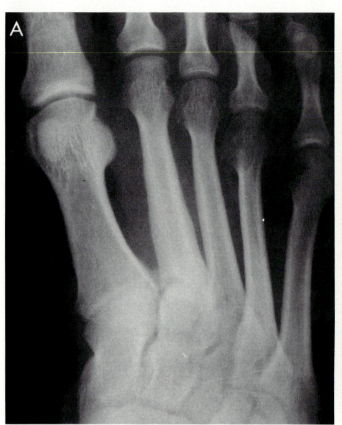
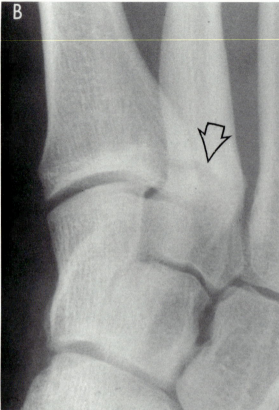

FIG 1–15.
A, Hyperostosis and uniform cortical thickening of the proximal two-thirds of the second metatarsal without a definite fracture line.
B (same patient as **A**), A coned view of the base of the second metatarsal demonstrates a stress fracture that extends completely across the metatarsal shaft *(arrow)*. (Permission for **A,B** granted courtesy of Pavlov H, Torg JS, Hersh A, et al: The roentgen examination of runners' injuries. *Radio-Graphics* 1981; 1:17–34.)

Metatarsal Stress Fracture—Complete

REMEDY Non-weight-bearing cast for 6 weeks or until radiographic and clinical healing occurs.

Stress Fracture—Base of the Fifth Metatarsal Distal to the Tuberosity

Fractures of the proximal part of the fifth metatarsal can be separated into two types: avulsion injuries involving the tuberosity, and fractures involving the proximal part of the diaphysis, distal to the tuberosity. Recently it has been recognized that the latter group, the Jones fracture, may be difficult to treat in the athlete. Note that successful treatment is dependent on accurate diagnosis of the fracture type, which may be (1) an acute fracture, (2) a fracture with a delayed union, or (3) a fracture with nonunion.

Acute Fracture

The distinguishing feature of an acute fracture is a narrow fracture line with short margins and no widening of the radiolucency, no intermedullary sclerosis, minimal cortical hypertrophy secondary to stress, and evidence of periosteal reaction.

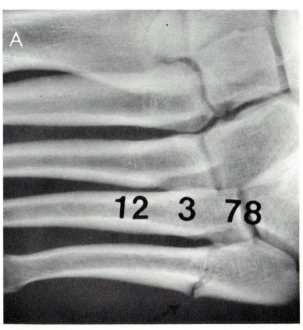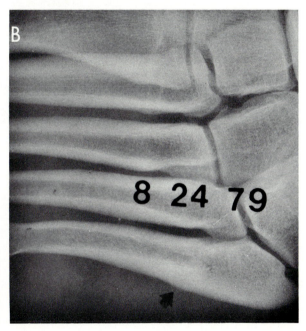

FIG 1–16.
A,B (both same patient), (12–3–78), There is a complete acute stress fracture of the fifth metatarsal distal to the tuberosity involving both cortices *(arrow)*. The fracture line is narrow without intermedullary sclerosis.
B (8–24–79), Complete healing *(arrow)* following 6 weeks in a non-weight-bearing toe-to-knee cast. (Permission for **A, B** granted courtesy of Torg JS, Balduini FC, Zelko RR, et al: Fractures of the base of the fifth metatarsal distal to the tuberosity. *J Bone Joint Surg* 1984; 66A:209–214.) *(Continued.)*

Delayed Union

The distinguishing features of a fracture with a delayed union are a history of previous injury or fracture, or both; a fracture line that involves both cortices with associated periosteal new bone; a widened line with adjacent radioluency due to bone resorption; and evidence of intermedullary sclerosis bordering the fracture margin.

FIG 1–16 (cont.).
C–E (all same patient), (9–6–77), Acute stress fracture distal to tuberosity *(arrow).* The fracture extends across the metatarsal shaft. The lateral cortex is thickened. *(Continued.)*

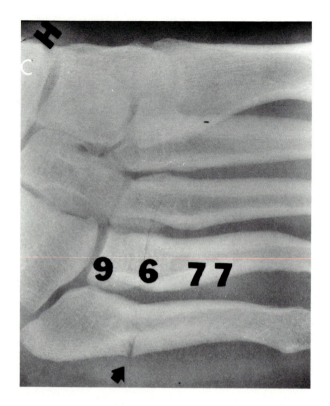

FIG 1–16 (cont.).
D (1–13–78), Four months later, the fracture line has widened and there is sclerosis along the fracture margins, partially obliterating the marrow cavity, indicating a delayed union.

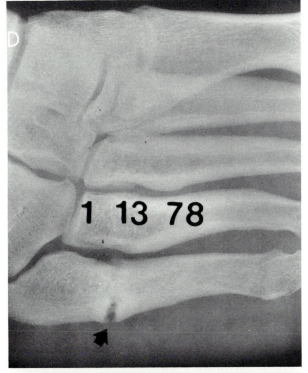

E (1–11–80), Two years later there is complete healing without surgery. (Permission for **C–E** granted courtesy of Torg JS, Balduini FC, Zelko RR, et al: Fractures of the base of the fifth metatarsal distal to the tuberosity. *J Bone Joint Surg* 1984; 66A:209–214.) *(Continued.)*

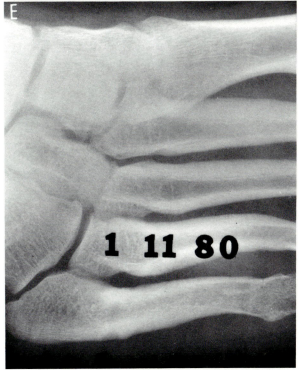

Delayed Union (cont.)

FIG 1–16 (cont.).
F–K (all same patient), (4–10–73), Initial radiograph demonstrated a radiolucent fracture line within an area of cortical hyperostosis in the inferior border of the fifth metatarsal, distal to the tuberosity. This was an incidental finding on films obtained for an ankle sprain.

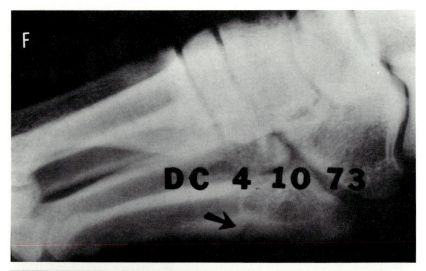

G (8–17–73), These x-rays were obtained following the acute onset of pain that occurred while the same patient was playing basketball. The fracture line has widened and there is intermedullary sclerosis, indicating a delayed union. The patient was placed in a weight-bearing cast for 2 weeks.

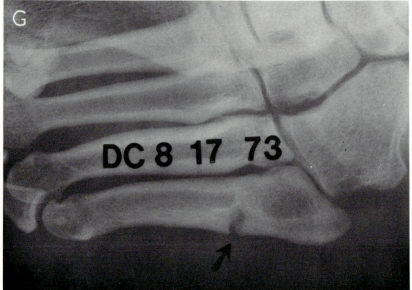

H (8–31–73), Follow-up x-rays demonstrate further widening of the fracture line. The patient was treated in a weight-bearing cast for 4 weeks, following which the patient returned to activity. (*Continued.*)

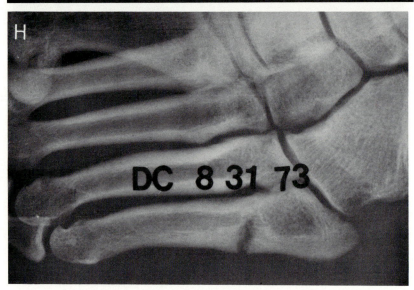

FIG 1–16 (cont.).
I (12–6–73), Progression of healing is identified radiographically but the fracture line is still evident. The patient was clinically healed.

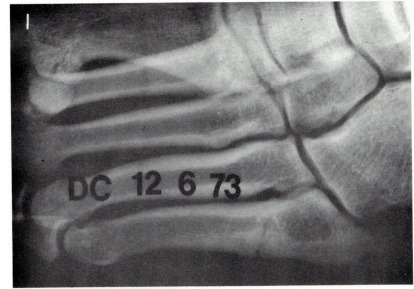

J (1–24–74), After return to activity, the patient reinjured himself and x-rays demonstrated widening of the fracture line.

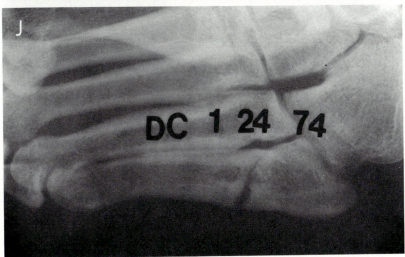

K (4–23–74), Three months following medullary curettage and an inlaid bone graft, there was complete incorporation of the bone graft. Healing occurred in 6 weeks. (Permission for **F,H** granted courtesy of Pavlov H, Torg JS, Hersh A, et al: The roentgen examination of runners' injuries. *RadioGraphics* 1981; 1:17–34.) *(Continued.)*

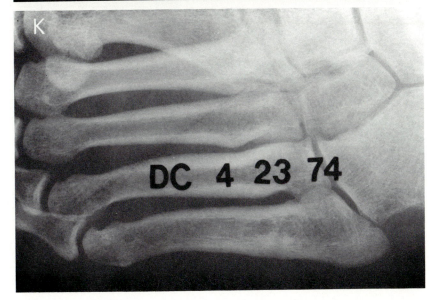

Nonunion

The features of a nonunion are a history of repetitive trauma and recurrent symptoms, a wide fracture line with periosteal new bone, and complete obliteration of the medullary cavity at the fracture site by sclerotic bone: the hallmark of a nonunion.

FIG 1–16 (cont.).
L, M (both same patient), (9–9–75), A stress fracture extends across the base of fifth metatarsal shaft, distal to tuberosity. The fracture margins are sclerotic with complete marrow obliteration, indicating a nonunion.

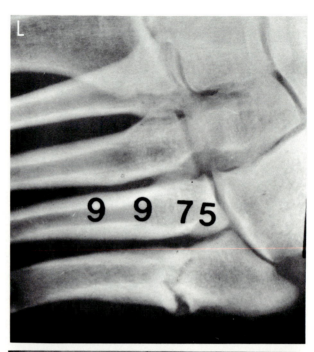

M (1–5–78), Follow-up x-rays for same patient as **L** two years following a medullary curettage and inlaid autogenous bone graft. There is no evidence of fracture.

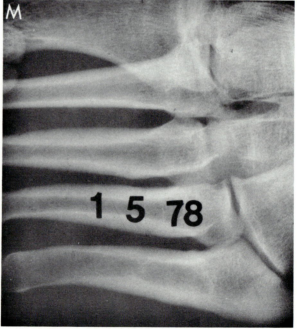

Metatarsal Stress Fracture—Base of the Fifth Metatarsal Distal to the Tuberosity

REMEDY

Acute fracture: non-weight-bearing cast for 6 weeks. *Delayed union:* if vigorous activity is avoided, healing occurs in a mean of 15 months. *Delayed union or a nonunion in the athlete:* a medullary curettage and inlaid bone graft is recommended. Examples of the surgical procedure is demonstrated in Figures **a** to **d**. The foot is immobilized in a non-weight-bearing toe-to-knee cast for 6 weeks. **a,** A rectangular piece of bone centered over the lateral aspect of the fracture is outlined with four drill holes. **b,** The piece of bone is excised with an osteotome. **c,** The sclerotic bone in the medullary canal is removed with a curet or drill, or both in order to reestablish the continuity of the medullary canal. **d,** An autogenous cortical bone graft, obtained from the anteromedial aspect of the distal part of the tibia, is carefully contoured with a high-speed bur and placed in the previously created defect. The periosteum, subcutaneous tissues, and skin are closed in layers. (Reference: Torg JS, Balduini FC, Zelko RR, et al: Fractures of the base of the fifth metatarsal distal to the tuberosity. *J Bone Joint Surg* 1984; 66A:209–214.)

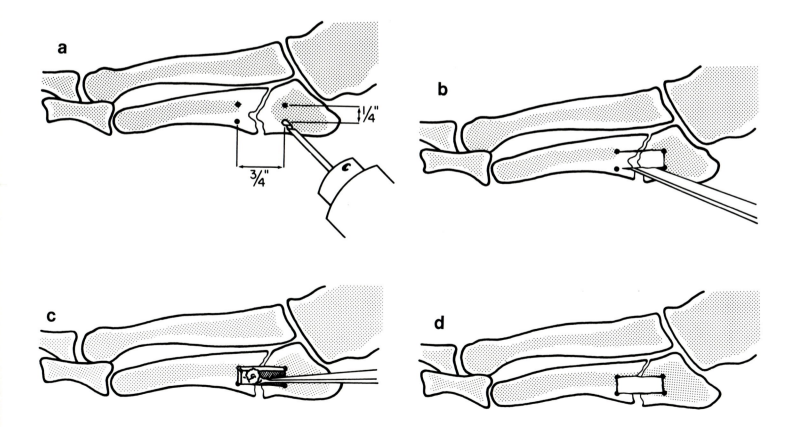

Metatarsal Stress Fracture—Delayed and/or Nonunion

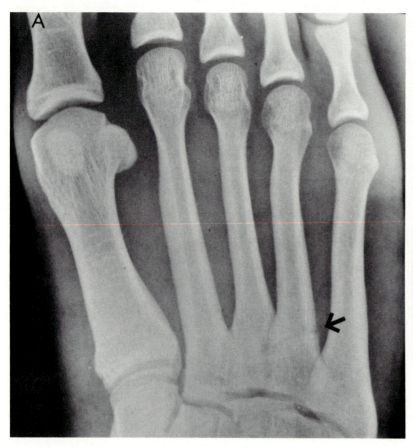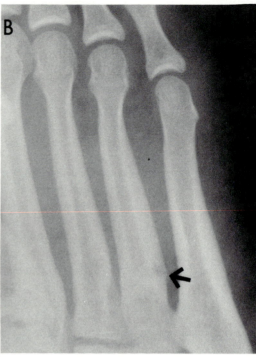

FIG 1–17.
A, Initial radiograph demonstrates faint periosteal new bone formation adjacent to the lateral aspect of the fourth metatarsal shaft (arrow).
B (same patient as **A**), Several months later the horizontal radiolucent fracture line persists (arrow). It is completely surrounded by sclerosis and is confined within the area of cortical hyperostosis indicating nonunion.

Metatarsal Stress Fracture—Delayed and/or Nonunion

REMEDY   This fracture behaves similarly to that occurring at the base of the fifth metatarsal distal to tuberosity and the same treatment principles apply.

Avulsion Injury—Fracture of the Tuberosity of the Fifth Metatarsal

Avulsion injuries of the base of fifth metatarsal are secondary to the insertion site of the peroneus brevis tendon. There are various patterns of this injury.

FIG 1–18.
A, Nondisplaced fracture fragments.

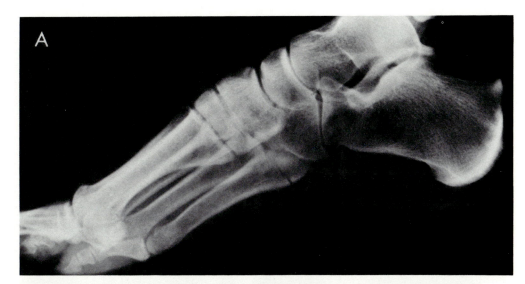

B, Slightly displaced fracture fragments.
C, Laterally displaced apophysis with adjacent soft tissue swelling. *(Continued.)*

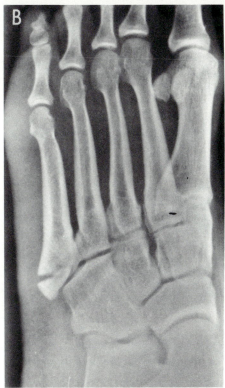
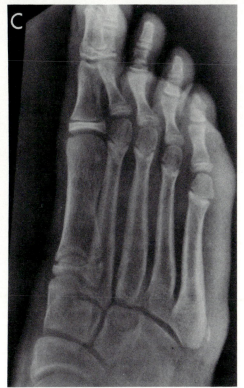

FIG 1–18 (cont.).
D, A horizontal fracture through the base of the right fifth metatarsal *(arrow)*. Normal, vertically oriented apophyseal centers are present bilaterally at the bases of the fifth metatarsals. (Permission for **D** granted courtesy of Pavlov H, Torg JS, Hersh A, et al: The roentgen examination of runners' injuries. *RadioGraphics* 1981; 1:17–34.)

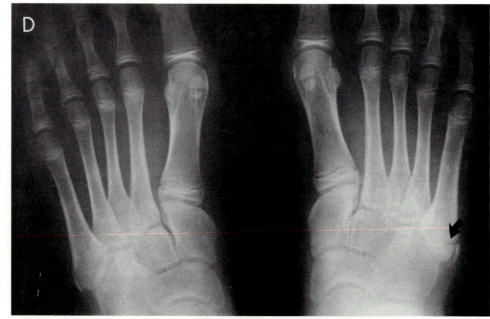

E, The horizontal fracture of the metatarsal base extends through the apophysis.

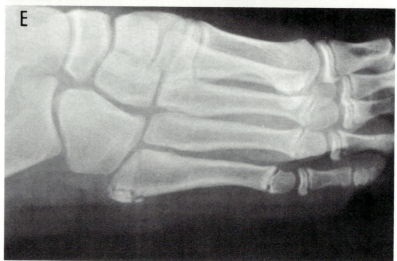

Avulsion Injury—Fracture of the Tuberosity of the Fifth Metatarsal

REMEDY   Activity restriction, rigid shoes, crutches as needed, protective strapping and padding until there is fracture union.

Necrosis—Freiberg's Infraction

Freiberg's infraction is an osteonecrosis of the second metatarsal head which is usually post-traumatic.

FIG 1–19.
The metatarsal head of the second metatarsal is flat and sclerotic. There is associated degenerative osteoarthritic changes at the metatarsal phalangeal joint.

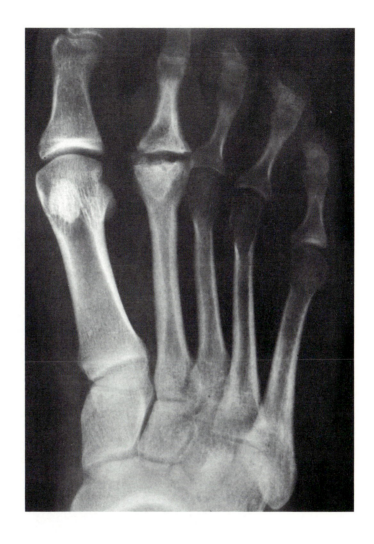

Necrosis—Freiberg's Infraction

REMEDY   *Adolescent:* conservative treatment with weight-bearing cast, followed by metatarsal pad. *Adult:* conservative treatment; if unresponsive, metatarsal head excision.

METATARSAL TARSAL JOINT

Juxta-articular Ossicles—Os Intermetatarseum

The os intermetatarseum is present on the dorsal aspect of the foot as a separate bone at the metatarsal tarsal joint, or attached to the base of the first or second metatarsal or the distal aspect of the first or second cuneiform.

FIG 1–20.
A, B (both same patient), Exostosis projects from the lateral and dorsal aspect of the first cuneiform *(arrow).*

C, Large exostosis projecting from the medial aspect of the base of the second metatarsal *(arrow).*

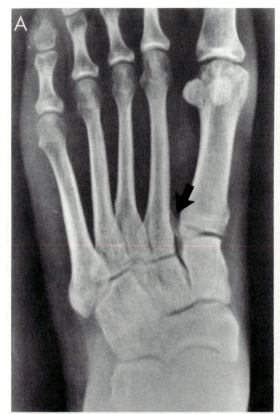

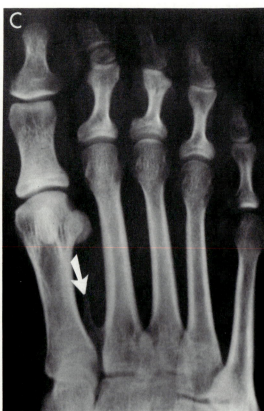

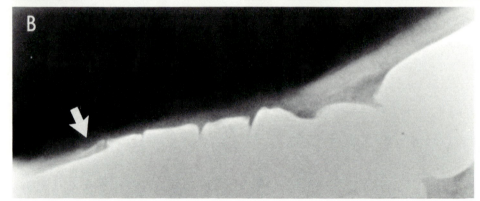

Juxta-articular Ossicles—Os Intermetatarseum

REMEDY   Orthotics or excision, if necessary.

**Metatarsal Tarsal Joint
Degenerative Osteoarthritis**

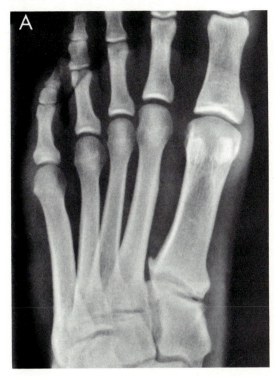

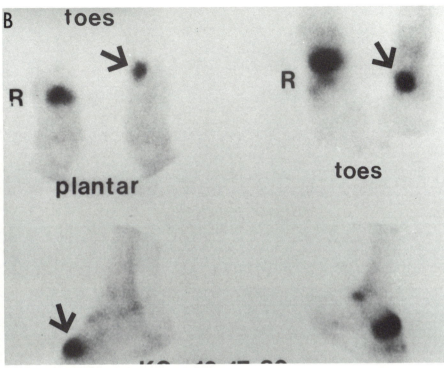

FIG 1–21.
A, Hypertrophic proliferative changes at the metatarsal tarsal joint of the first digit.

B (same patient as **A**), Clockwise: plantar, frontal, right and left lateral. The radionuclide bone scan of the left foot demonstrates localized augmented uptake corresponding to x-ray findings *(arrows)*. Note: the uptake in the right foot is secondary to a navicular stress fracture and will be discussed later.

**Metatarsal Tarsal Joint
Degenerative Osteoarthritis**

REMEDY   Orthotics, aspirin, and activity restriction.

NAVICULAR

Juxta-articular Ossicles

There are two juxta-articular ossicles associated with the navicular: the os tibialis externa, medially; and the os supranaviculare, dorsally.

FIG 1–22.
Os Tibialis Externa (Accessory Navicular)
A, A normal asymptomatic os tibialis externa is a well corticated triangular osseous density proximal to the medial tuberosity of the navicular. The ossicle borders are corticated and beveled and the ossicle does not "fit" together with the navicular.

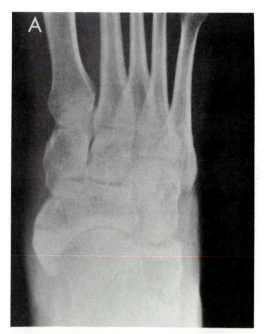

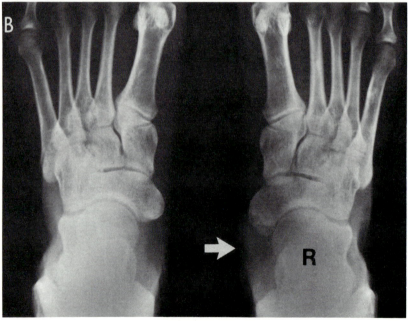

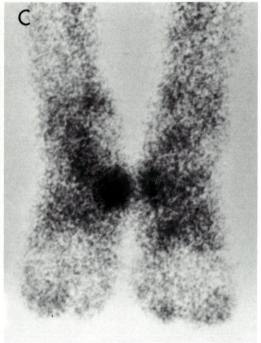

B, Os tibialis externa on the right *(R)* is symptomatic; the adjacent soft tissues are swollen *(arrow).*
C (same patient as **B**), A radionuclide bone scan of both feet demonstrates augmented isotope uptake localized to the right os tibialis externa. The isotope uptake confirms increased bone production secondary to motion between the bone fragments. *(Continued.)*

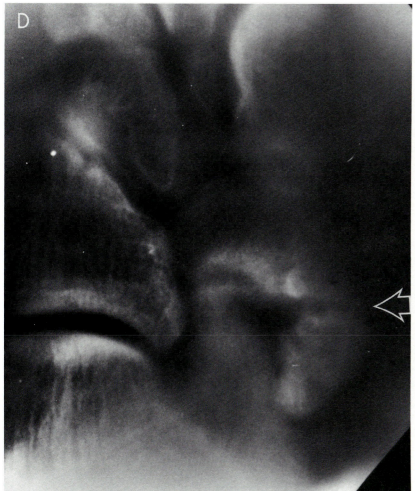

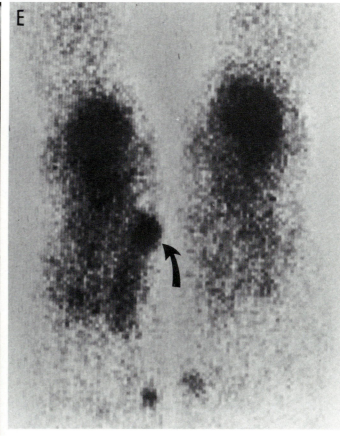

FIG 1–22 (cont.).
D, E (both same patient), A tomogram of a symptomatic os tibialis externa demonstrates a pseudoarthrosis between the os tibialis externa and the navicular. A pseudoarthrosis is evidenced by irregular and sclerotic borders.
E, On the radionuclide bone scan, localized augmented isotope uptake *(arrow)* confirms motion and bone production at this site.

Juxta-articular Ossicles

Os Tibialis Externa (Accessory Navicular)

REMEDY   If symptomatic, longitudinal arch supports; possible excision of accessory fragment.

Os Supranaviculare

FIG 1–23.
A–C, Three examples: the os supranaviculare is located at the proximal dorsal navicular border *(arrow)*. It does not "fit" with the adjacent bone. The margins of the bone are corticated and beveled. There are various shapes and sizes. *(Continued.)*

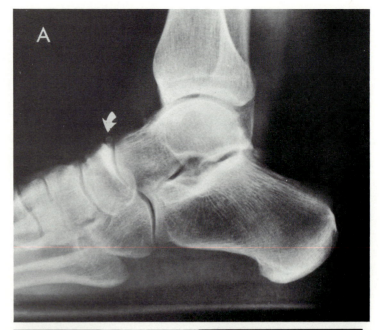

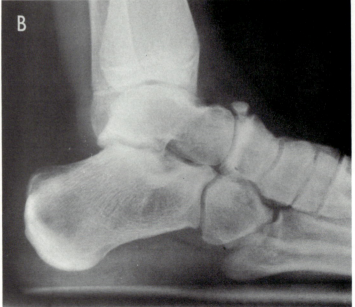

FIG 1–23 (cont.).

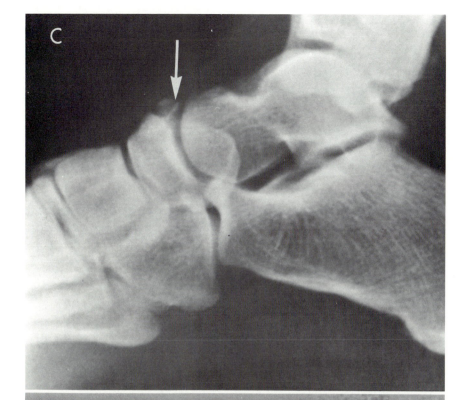

D (same patient as **C**), Localized augmented isotope uptake at the proximal dorsal aspect of the navicular on a radionuclide bone scan confirms abnormal motion at this site *(arrow)*. Incidentally, this patient also has uptake at the plantar fascial insertion site onto the calcaneus indicating calcific fasciitis.

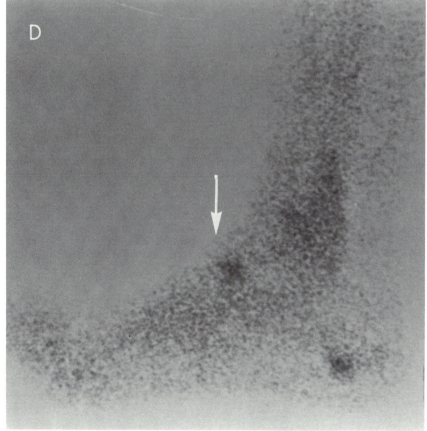

(See Remedy on following page.)

Juxta-articular Ossicles

Os Supranaviculare

REMEDY   Conservative treatment. If symptoms are unresponsive, excision of the ossicle.

Avulsion Injury—Navicular

FIG 1–24.
A small avulsion fracture *(closed arrow)* from the proximal navicular with swelling and increased radiodensity of the adjacent soft tissue *(open arrow)*.

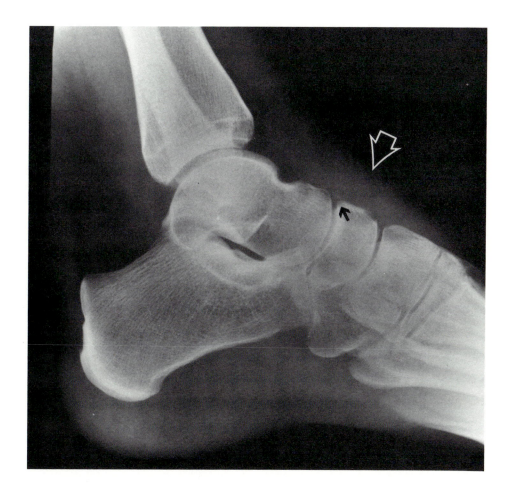

Avulsion Injury—Navicular

REMEDY   Ice, wrap, and crutches as needed.

Stress Fracture—Navicular—Partial

A partial fracture of the navicular is confined within the dorsal surface and involves the proximal articular border, the distal articular border or both.

FIG 1–25.
A, Anatomic AP tomogram through the dorsal surface of the bone demonstrates a partial stress fracture of the proximal articular border.

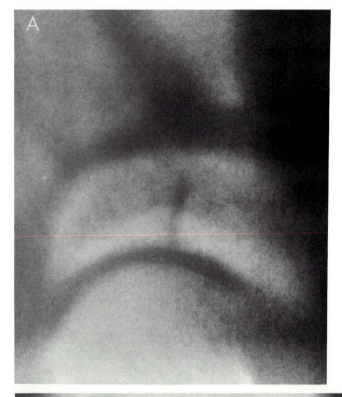

B, Anatomic AP tomogram through the dorsal surface of the bone demonstrates a partial stress fracture involving the distal articular border. *(Continued.)*

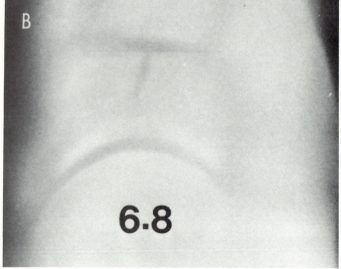

FIG 1–25 (cont.).
C, Anatomic AP tomogram through dorsal surface of bone demonstrates partial stress fracture of the proximal articular border (*arrow*) combined with a transverse fracture fragment within the medial aspect of the talonavicular joint.

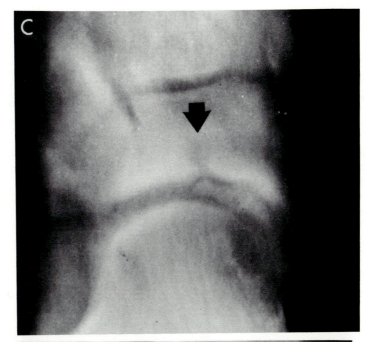

D, Anatomic AP tomogram through dorsal surface of bone demonstrates partial fracture extending from the proximal to distal articular borders, but, as demonstrated by tomography, the fracture is confined within the dorsal surface of the bone. (*Continued.*)

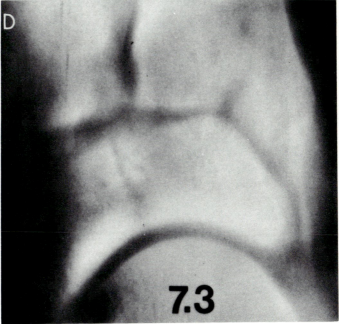

**Stress Fracture—Navicular—
Partial (cont.)**

FIG 1–25 (cont.).
E, Lateral tomogram demonstrates a
transverse fracture in the proximal articular surface with a dorsal fragment
(*arrowhead*) and an intramedullary
cyst (*arrow*).

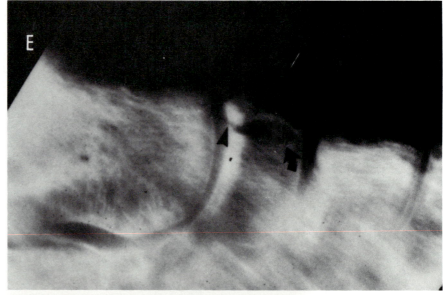

F, Axial computed tomogram (CT) image of the navicular demonstrates the
partial fracture confined to the dorsal
aspect of the navicular. (*Continued.*)

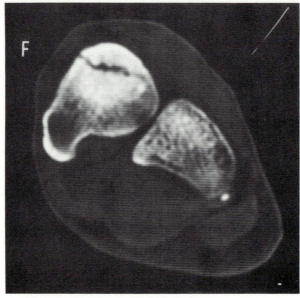

FIG 1–25 (cont.).

G,H (both same patient), Para-axial reformatted CT images demonstrate partial fractures in the sagittal plane that involve the proximal articular border. The fracture of the left foot is an acute fracture *(arrow)*, while that on the right is a chronic fracture with sclerotic margins. (Permission for **A, D** granted courtesy of Pavlov H, Torg JS, Freiberger RH: Tarsal navicular fractures: Radiographic evaluation. *Radiology* 1983; 148:641. Permission for **B, C, E** granted courtesy of Torg JS, Pavlov H, Cooley L, et al: Stress fractures of the tarsal navicular. A retrospective review of twenty-one cases. *J Bone Joint Surg* 1982; 63A:700.)

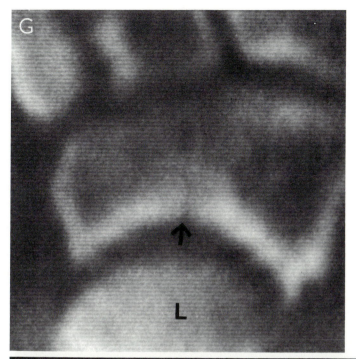

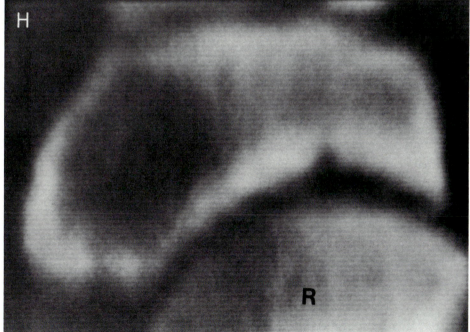

Stress Fracture—Navicular—Partial

REMEDY   Non-weight-bearing cast 6 to 8 weeks.

Stress Fracture—Navicular—Complete

A complete navicular fracture involves the proximal and distal articular borders and extends completely through the bone.

FIG 1–26.
A, Routine anteroposterior (AP) view of the foot demonstrates a complete sagittal fracture *(arrow)*. The fracture may be overlooked if the tarsal area is underpenetrated or if the lateral fragment is misinterpreted as a separate tarsal bone. *(Continued.)*

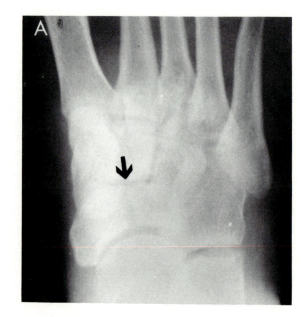

FIG 1–26 (cont.).
B, Routine AP view of the foot demonstrates the sagittal fracture *(arrow)*. The fracture may be overlooked if the lateral fragment is misinterpreted as a separate tarsal bone.

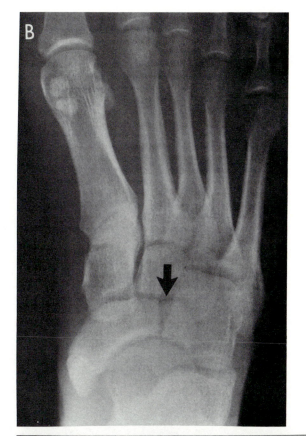

C (same patient as **B**), An anatomic AP tomogram demonstrates a complete sagittal tarsal navicular stress fracture. Incidentally, there is an asymptomatic os tibialis externa. (Permission for **C** granted courtesy of Torg JS, Pavlov H, Cooley L, et al: Stress fractures of the tarsal navicular. A retrospective review of twenty-one cases. *J Bone Joint Surg* 1982; 63A:700.) *(Continued.)*

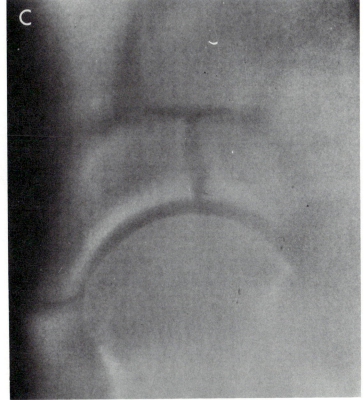

Stress Fracture—Navicular—Complete (cont.)

FIG 1–26 (cont.).
D–G (all same patient), Routine views of the foot demonstrate a complete tarsal navicular stress fracture on the left *(arrow)*.

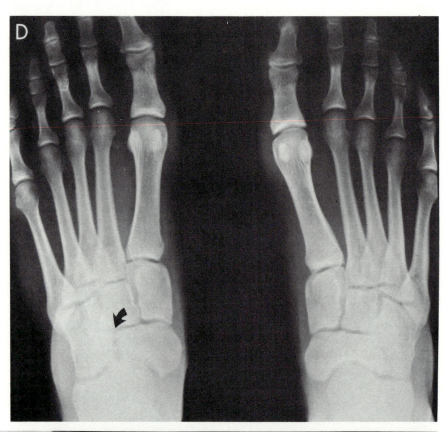

E, On a lateral view of the foot, obtained with the patient standing, there is malalignment of the dorsal surfaces of the navicular and cuneiforms which is commonly present in these patients. *(Continued.)*

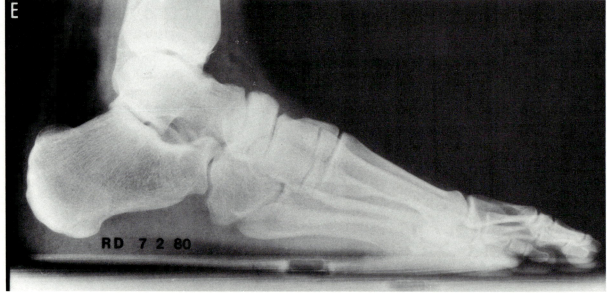

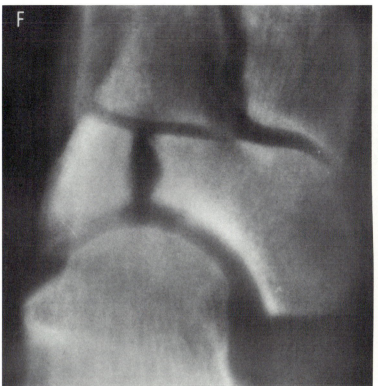

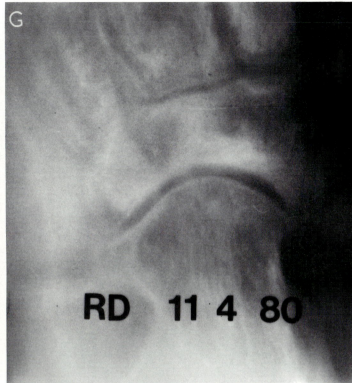

FIG 1–26 (cont.).

F (same patient as **D, E**), The tarsal navicular fracture is best demonstrated on an anatomic AP tomogram. In this patient, the fracture margins are sclerotic and there is complete obliteration of the marrow cavity, indicating a nonunion. The medial fragment is medially displaced and the entire lateral fragment is "white" or radiodense, indicating avascular necrosis.

G (same patient), On a tomogram obtained following medullary curettage and inlaid autogenous bone graft, complete incorporation and healing is demonstrated. (Permission for **D, E** granted courtesy of Pavlov H, Torg JS, Freiberger RH: Tarsal navicular fractures: Radiographic evaluation. *Radiology* 1983; 148:641. Permission for **F, G** granted courtesy of Torg JS, Pavlov H, Cooley L, et al: Stress fractures of the tarsal navicular. A retrospective review of twenty-one cases. *J Bone Joint Surg* 1982; 63A:700.)

Stress Fracture—Navicular—Complete

REMEDY

Acute or delayed union: non-weight-bearing cast for 6 to 8 weeks. *Nonunion:* medullary curettage and autogenous bone graft as demonstrated in **a** to **f**.

a, Diagram of a navicular nonunion. **b,** A rectangular piece of bone centered over the sagittal fracture is outlined with four drill holes. **c,** The piece of bone is excised with an osteotome. **d, e,** The sclerotic bone in the medullary canal is removed with a curet or drill or both. **f,** An autogenous cortical bone graft is placed in the created defect.

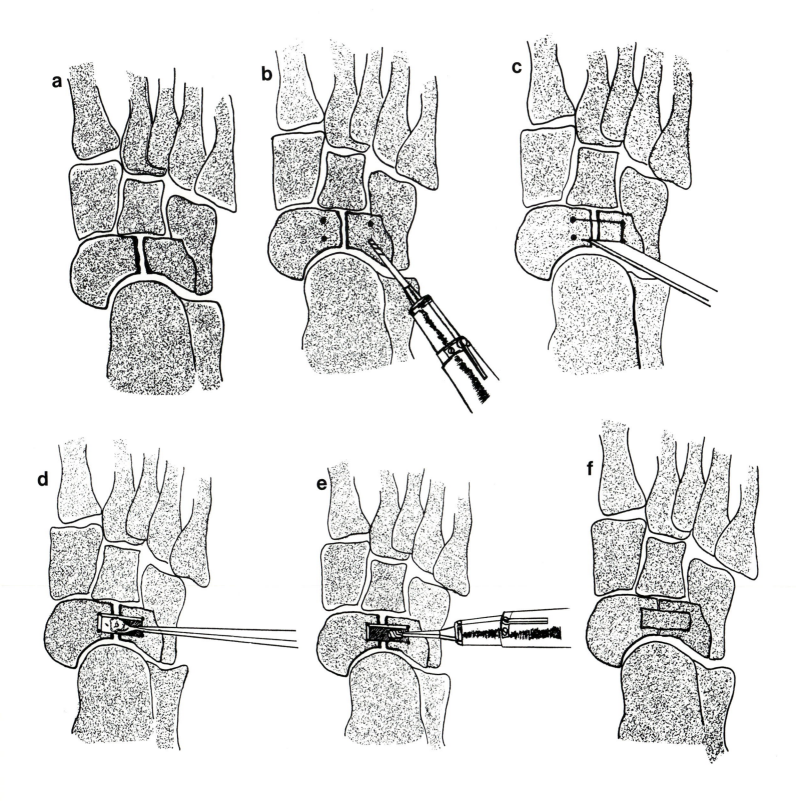

Technique for Roentgen Evaluation of Tarsal Navicular Injuries

Radionuclide Bone Scan

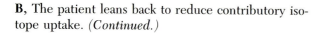

FIG 1–27.

A, Early detection of stress fractures is made by a bone scan. Optimal visualization is with the plantar view obtained by placing the soles of the feet flat on the face of the gamma camera.

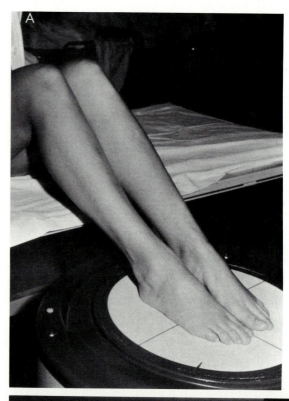

B, The patient leans back to reduce contributory isotope uptake. *(Continued.)*

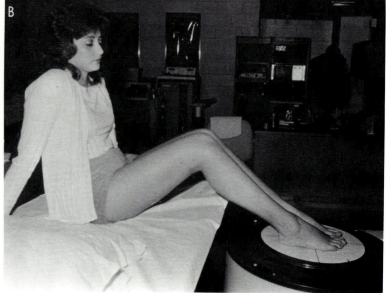

FIG 1–27 (cont.).

C, The plantar view *(right lower corner)*, best demonstrates localized augmented uptake confined to the navicular. On the plantar view, the uptake has the configuration of the navicular. On the usual frontal view, obtained with the camera on the dorsal surface of the feet *(left upper corner)*, the uptake from the hindfoot is superimposed on the midfoot. Incidentally, the patient also has a stress fracture of the third left metatarsal shaft. (Permission for **C** granted courtesy of Pavlov H, Torg JS, Freiberger RH: Tarsal navicular fractures: Radiographic evaluation. *Radiology* 1983; 148:641.) *(Continued.)*

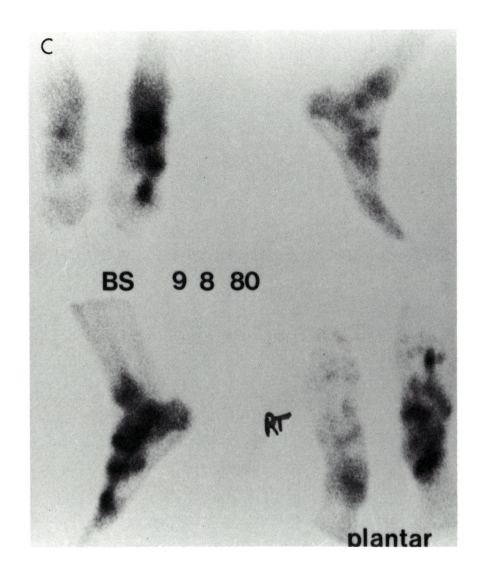

Anatomic AP Tomograms

Partial stress fractures are confined within the dorsal surface and are demonstrated on a tomogram obtained through the most dorsal aspect of the midthird of the navicular. The anatomic AP tomogram of the navicular is performed with the forefoot resting on a sponge so it is elevated and supinated slightly. The anatomic AP position is necessary because it is essential that the dorsal surface of the navicular be parallel to the tabletop and the plane of the tomogram. Also, the entire middle third of the navicular must be seen en face.

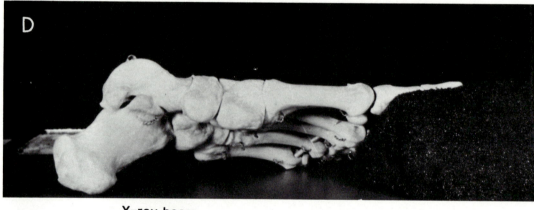

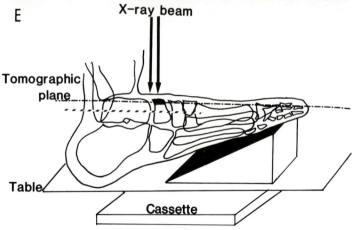

FIG 1–27 (cont.)
D, E, The position of the foot for the anatomic AP position is compared to that of the usual foot position (**F, G**) via skeleton models and diagrams. Note that for the anatomic AP position (**D, E**), the dorsal aspect of the navicular is parallel to the plane of the tomogram. The *shaded area* on the diagrams demonstrates that area in which these fractures occur. (Permission for **D, F** granted courtesy of Torg JS, Pavlov H, Cooley L, et al: Stress fractures of the tarsal navicular. A retrospective review of twenty-one cases. *J Bone Joint Surg* 1982; 63A:700.)

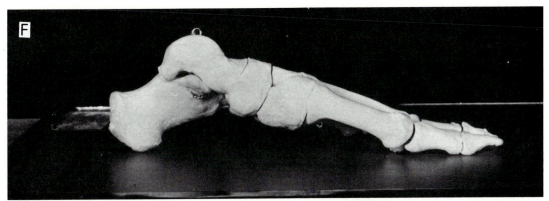

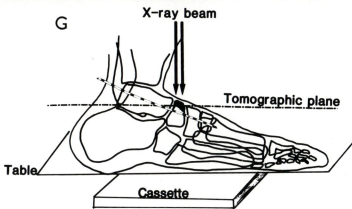

Osteoid Osteoma of the Navicular

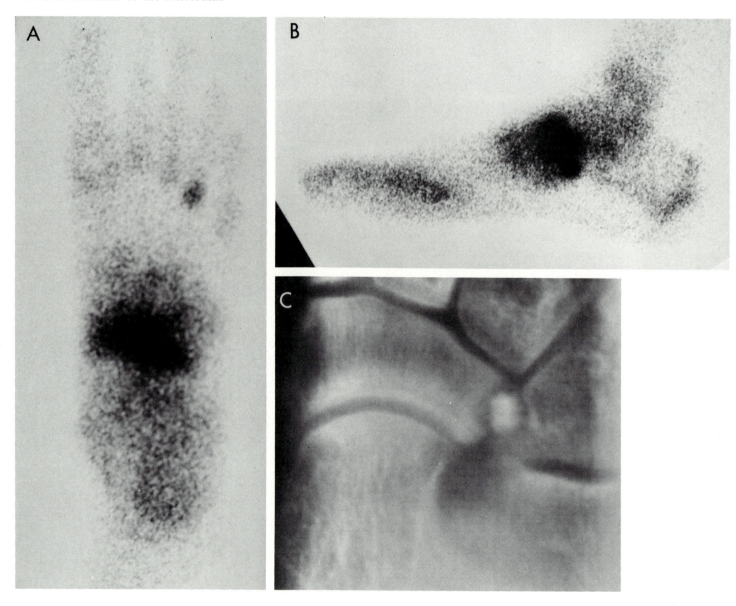

FIG 1–28.
A, B, C (all same patient), Augmented radionuclide uptake in
the navicular simulates the uptake seen with a stress fracture,
except that on the lateral view (**B**) there is a separate area of
uptake near the plantar aspect. On the oblique view of the foot
(**C**), the sclerotic nidus of the osteoid osteoma is identified in
the lateral aspect of the navicular.

Osteoid Osteoma of the Navicular

REMEDY   Surgical excision.

Necrosis—Köhler's Disease

FIG 1–29.

A dense, small, irregularly contoured navicular can be normal if the child is asymptomatic. (Ref: Köhler A.: Uber eine haufige bisher ansch unbetannte erkranlung einzelner kindlicher knochen. *Munchen Med Uschr* 1908; 55:1923.)

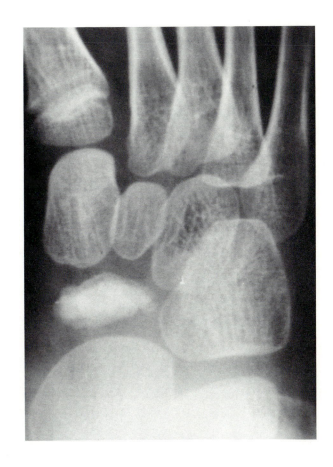

Necrosis—Köhler's Disease

REMEDY   *Mild or minimal pain:* longitudinal arch support. *Severe pain:* short leg walking cast.

TALUS

Juxta-articular Ossicles

There are two juxta-articular ossicles associated with talus, the os supratalare, superiorly, and the os trigonum, posteriorly.

Os Supratalare

The os supratalare is located dorsal to the waist of the talus. The margins are corticated and beveled. Note the proximity of the ossicle to the anterior tibial lip when the foot is in dorsiflexion.

FIG 1–30.
A, This patient has a large os supratalare and a degenerative spur dorsal to the navicular. Incidentally, this patient also has calcification in the plantar fascia. *(Continued.)*

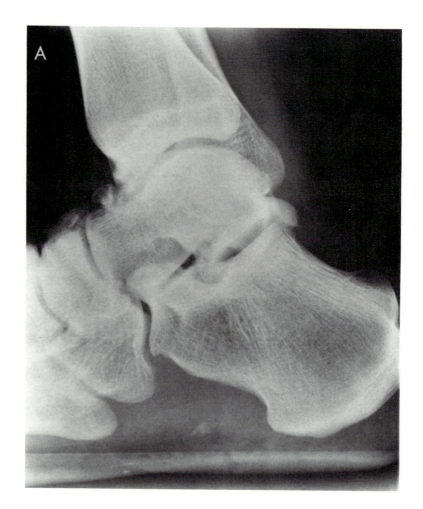

FIG 1–30 (cont.).
B, Large, well-corticated ossicle at the dorsal aspect of talus. The ossicle is attempting articulation with the talus, and a fibrous or cartilaginous union cannot be excluded.

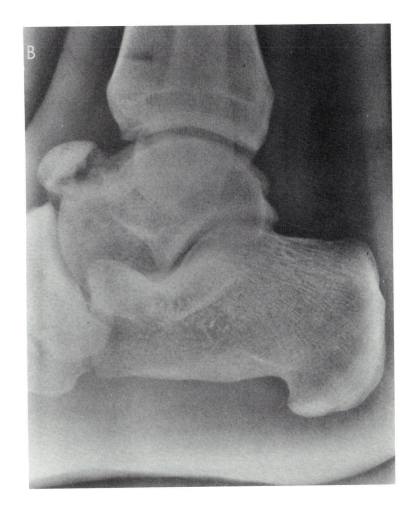

Juxta-articular Ossicles

Os Supratalare

REMEDY   Conservative treatment with excision of the ossicle if symptoms are unresponsive.

Os Trigonum

The os trigonum is located at the posterior process of the talus. An os trigonum can be present with a long posterior talar process (Stieda's process). The ossicle margins are corticated and slightly beveled and the ossicle does not "fit" precisely with the talus.

FIG 1–31.
A–C, Os trigonums vary in shape and size. Three examples. (Permission for **B** granted courtesy of Pavlov H, Torg JS, Hersh A, et al: The roentgen examination of runners' injuries. *RadioGraphics* 1981; 1:17–34.)

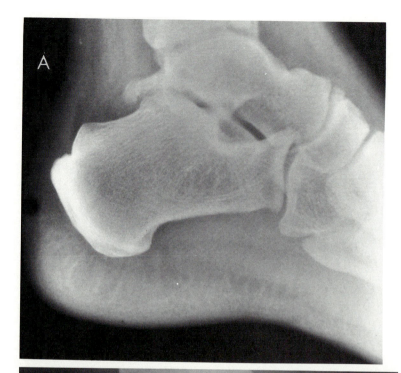

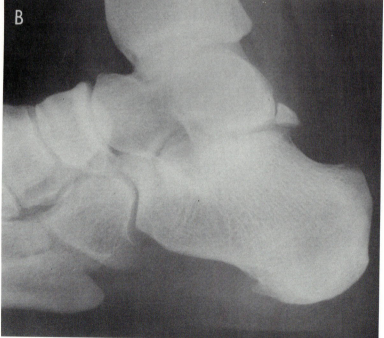

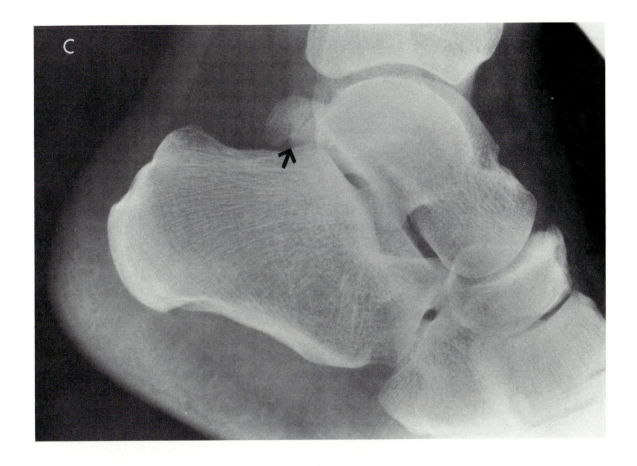

Juxta-articular Ossicles

Os Trigonum

REMEDY   Rehabilitation exercises and excision if symptoms are unresponsive.

Avulsion Injury—Talus

FIG 1–32.
A, Avulsion fracture from the dorsal aspect of the distal talus.

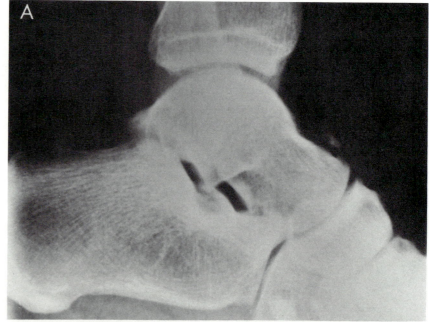

B, Avulsion fracture from the midtalus with adjacent soft tissue swelling.

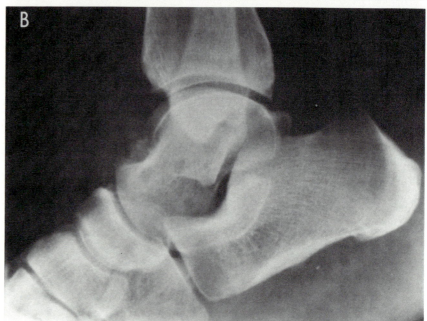

Avulsion Injury—Talus

REMEDY   Ice, wrap, and crutches as needed.

Fracture—Posterior Talar Process

Fracture of the posterior talar process is usually secondary to extreme plantar flexion in which the posterior talar tubercle is wedged between the calcaneus and the posterior rim of the tibia.

FIG 1–33.

A, B (both same patient), A faint radiolucent line *(arrow)* at the posterior aspect of the talus is most consistent with an os trigonum; however, a follow-up radiograph, 10 days later, **B,** demonstrates widening of the radiolucent line indicating resorption along the fracture margins and healing. (Permission for **B** granted courtesy of Pavlov H, Torg JS, Hersh A, et al: The roentgen examination of runners' injuries. *RadioGraphics* 1981; 1:17–34.) *(Continued.)*

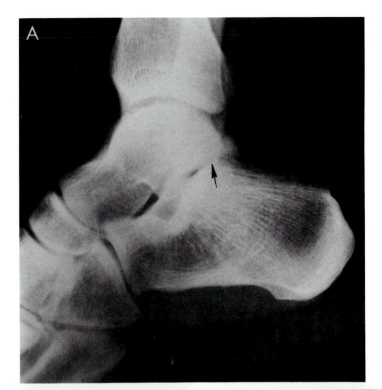

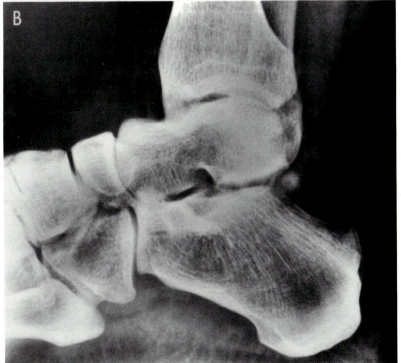

Fracture—Posterior Talar Process (cont.)

FIG 1–33 (cont.).
C, An acute radiolucent fracture line (*arrow*) separates the posterior fragment from the talus. The fragments fit together and there is no sclerosis bordering the fracture margins. (*Continued.*)

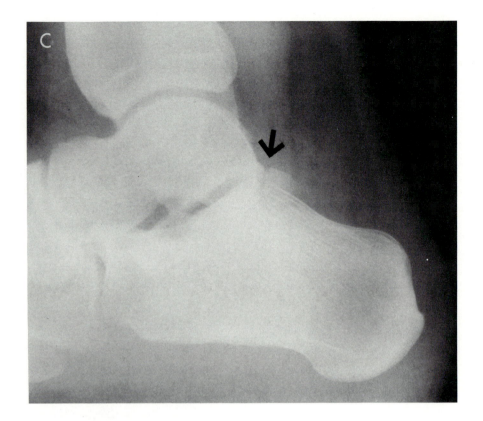

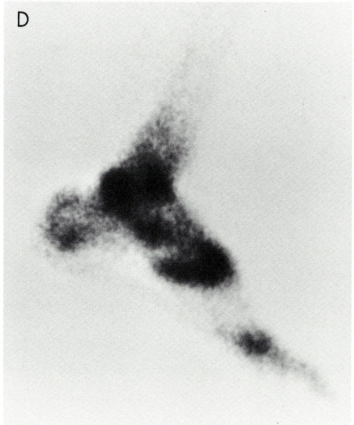

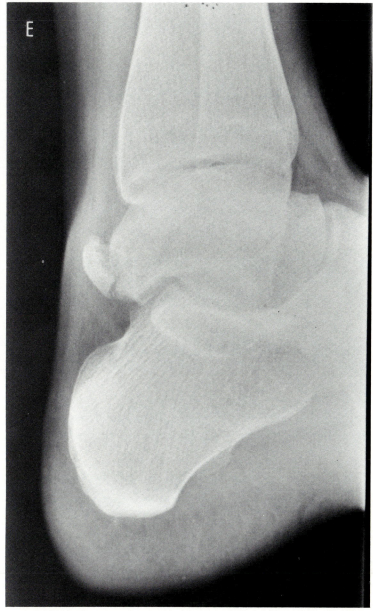

FIG 1–33 (cont.).
D, E (both same patient), A radionuclide bone scan demonstrates augmented isotope uptake in the posterior talus and a slightly external oblique view of the talus, **E**, demonstrates the fracture. The increased radiodensity of the adjacent soft tissues indicates inflammation. (*Continued.*)

Fracture—Posterior Talar Process (cont.)

FIG 1–33 (cont.).
F–I (all same patient), A fracture of the posterior talar process is present at the initial presentation. *(Continued.)*

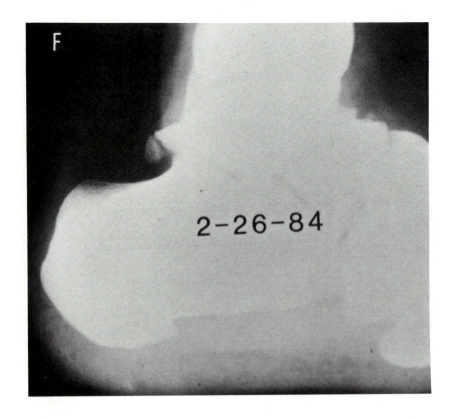

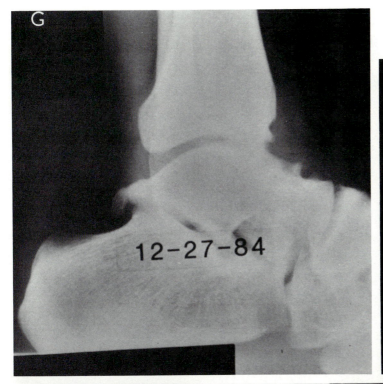

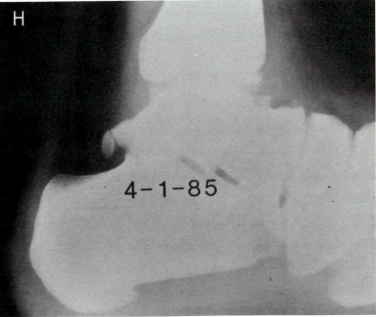

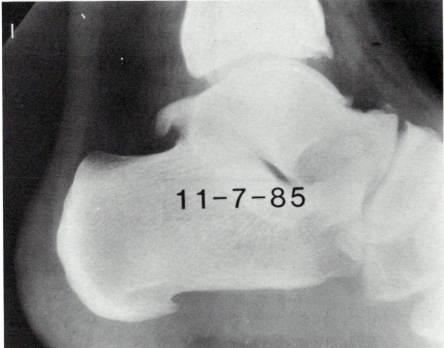

FIG 1–33 (cont.).
G, At examination 10 months later, the fracture healed.
H, Following repeat trauma, the posterior process refractured and, **I,** the fracture again healed.

Fracture—Posterior Talar Process

REMEDY   For a single episode, nonweight-bearing crutches, followed by ankle rehabilitation exercises. With repeat episodes of fracture, surgical excision of posterior talar process is recommended.

SUBTALAR JOINT

Sustentacular Coalition

Routine Radiograph

FIG 1–34.
A, B, A tarsal coalition is suggested on the routine x-rays by a bulbus projection along the dorsal surface of the waist of talus without congruent deformity of the navicular. (Permission for **A** granted courtesy of Goldman AB, Pavlov H, Schneider R: Radionuclide bone scanning in subtalar coalitions: Differential considerations. *Am J Roentgenol* 1982; 138:427.) *(Continued.)*

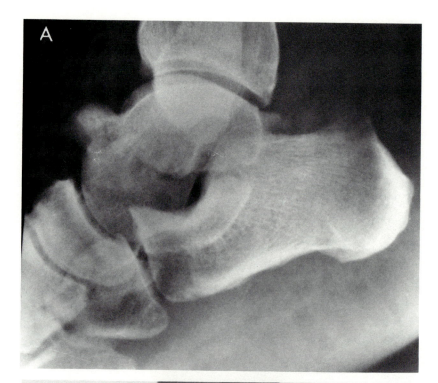

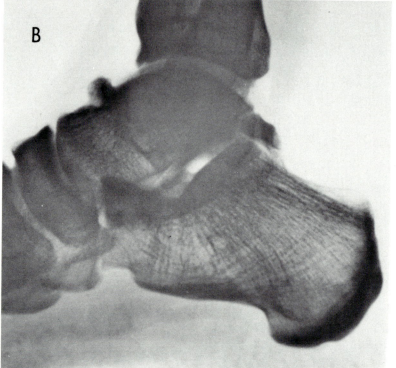

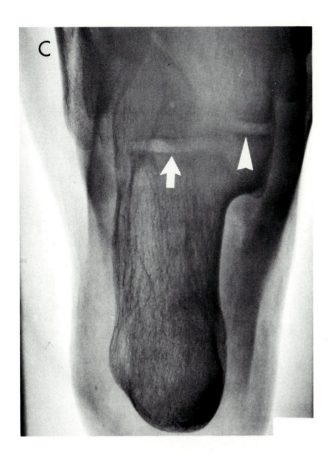

FIG 1–34 (cont.).
C, On the Harris view, the normal sustentacular and posterior compartments of the subtalar joint are oriented perpendicular to the longitudinal axis of the calcaneus. The sustentacular joint is medial *(arrowhead)* and the posterior subtalar joint is lateral *(arrow);* both joint compartments are of equal width with intact articular cortical margins. *(Continued.)*

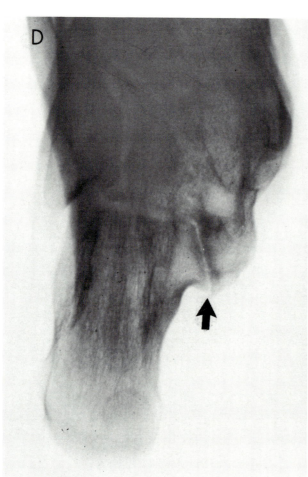

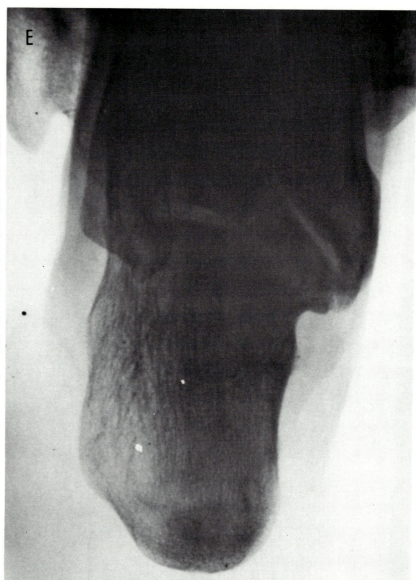

Sustentacular Coalition (cont.)

FIG 1–34 (cont.).
D, E, A fibrous or cartilaginous coalition of
a sustentacular joint with degenerative osteoarthritic changes *(arrow)* is identified on
the Harris view by its oblique orientation
(almost parallel to the axis of the calcaneus).
The articular surfaces are irregular and the
joint compartment is narrowed. *(Continued.)*

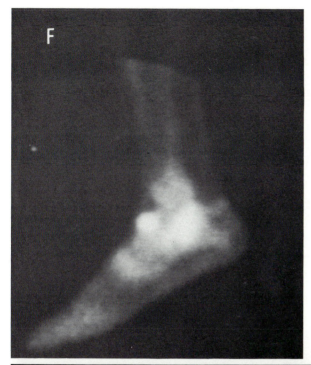

Radionuclide Bone Scan

FIG 1–34 (cont.).

F (same patient as **A**), **G** (same patient as **B**), A sustentacular coalition is demonstrated on radionuclide bone scan by augmented isotope uptake in the region of the talar beak and in the posterior subtalar joint; the augmented isotope uptake corresponds to the sites of bony proliferation on the talus and abnormal motion. There is no abnormal uptake at the site of a complete bony coalition. (Permission for **F** granted courtesy of Goldman AB, Pavlov H, Schneider R: Radionuclide bone scanning in subtalar coalitions: Differential consideration. *Am J Roentgenol* 1982; 138:427.) (*Continued.*)

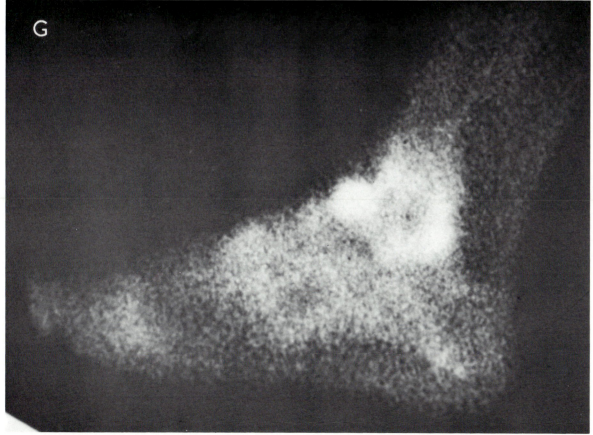

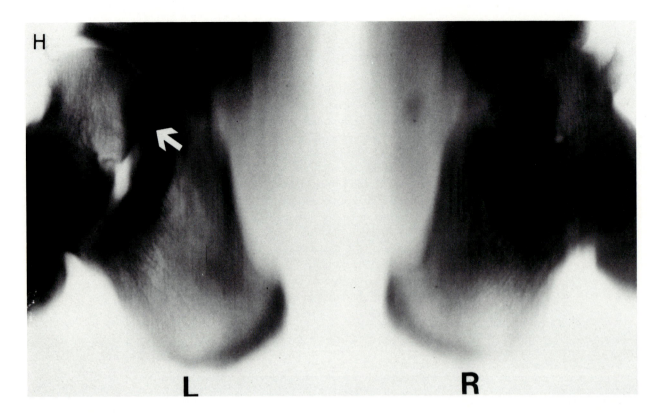

Sustentacular Coalition (cont.)

Tomogram

FIG 1–34 (cont.).
H (same patient as **A** and **F**), A lateral tomogram of both feet demonstrates the talar
beak on the right and a complete osseous
fusion of the sustentacular joint. The normal sustentacular joint *(arrow)* is seen on
the left. (Permission for **H** granted courtesy
of Goldman AB, Pavlov H, Schneider R:
Radionuclide bone scanning in subtalar coalitions: Differential considerations. *Am J
Roentgenol* 1982; 138:427.) *(Continued.)*

Arthrogram

FIG 1–34 (cont.).
I, J, Following the injection of contrast into the talonavicular joint, contrast normally communicates with the sustentacular joint and is demonstrated on the lateral (**I**) or Harris views (**J**). With a sustentacular coalition, contrast injected into the talonavicular joint is confined to the talonavicular joint (**K**) and indicates a fibrous or cartilaginous coalition. (Permission for **K** granted courtesy of Pavlov H: Ankle and subtalar arthrography. In Symposium of Ankle and Foot Problems in the Athlete. *Clin Sports Med* 1982; 1:47–69.) *(Continued.)*

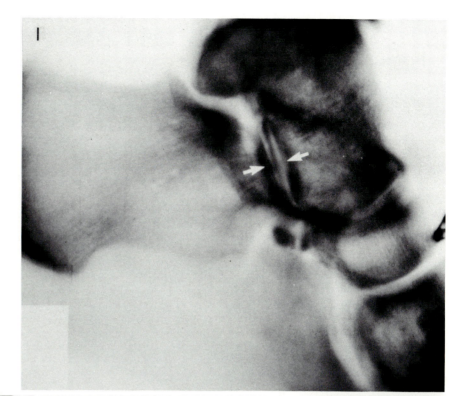

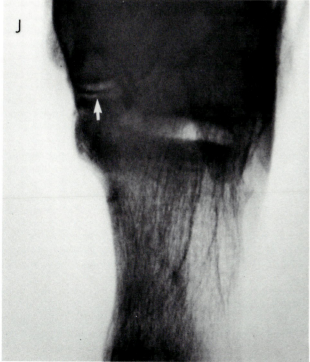

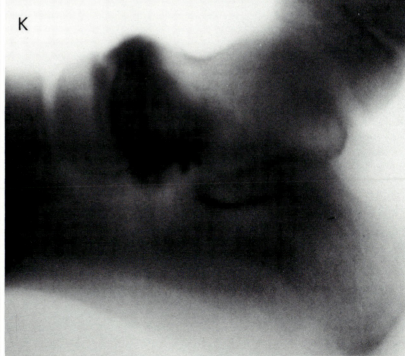

Sustentacular Coalition (cont.)

CT Scan

FIG 1–34 (cont.).
L, CT scan through subtalar joints demonstrates bilateral fibrous or cartilaginous sustentacular coalitions with degenerative osteoarthritic changes.

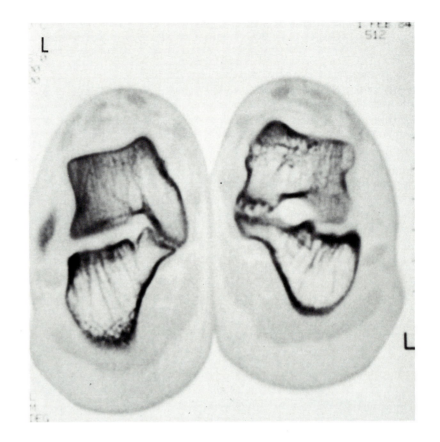

Sustentacular Coalition

REMEDY   Conservative management consists of non-weight-bearing cast, activity limitation and orthotics. If symptoms become disabling, triple arthrodesis.

Posterior Subtalar Joint Osteoarthritis

FIG 1–35.
Degenerative osteoarthritis of the posterior
subtalar joint *(arrow)* with hypertrophic
spurs, joint narrowing, and sclerosis along
the articular margins. (Permission granted
courtesy of Pavlov H: Ankle and subtalar
arthrography. In Symposium of Ankle and
Foot Problems in the Athlete. *Clin Sports
Med* 1982; 1:47–69.)

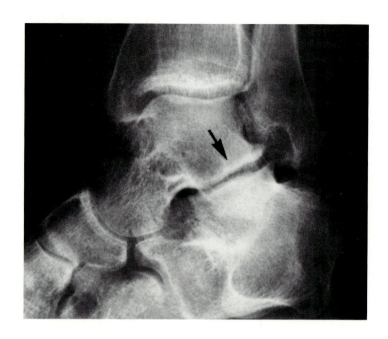

Posterior Subtalar Joint Osteoarthritis

REMEDY   Local symptoms may respond to shoe and activity modification
and/or steroid injection. Degenerative osteoarthritis that occurs
in an unusual site, however, suggests underlying systemic con-
ditions such as calcium pyrophosphate deposition disease
(CPPD) or pseudogout, and a systemic disease process should
be excluded.

CUBOID

Juxta-articular Ossicles—Os Peroneum

FIG 1–36.
A–D, These ossicles are located at the calcaneal cuboid joint. They vary in shape and size and can be bipartite.

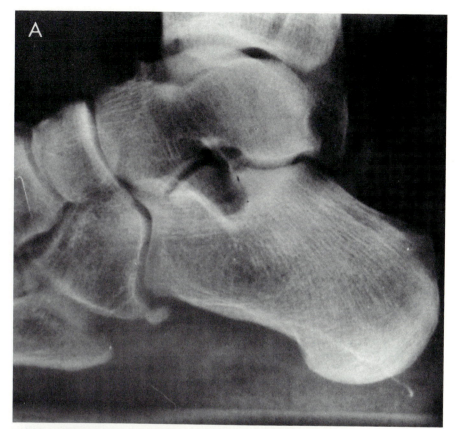

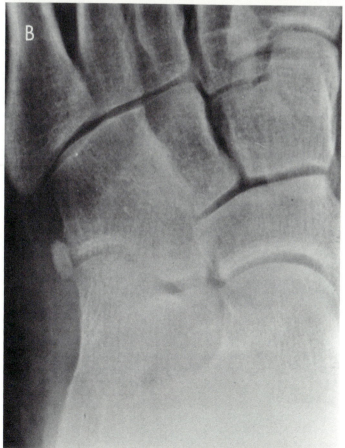

(Figures C,D appear on following page.)

Juxta-articular Ossicles—Os Peroneum (cont.)

FIG 1–36 (cont.).

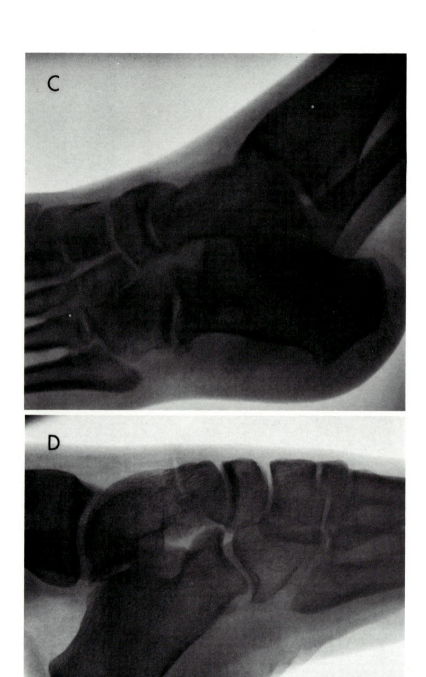

Juxta-articular Ossicles—Os Peroneum

REMEDY If symptomatic, steroid injection.

Stress Fracture—Cuboid

FIG 1–37.
A, B (both same patient), Tomogram through the cuboid demonstrates a radiolucent fracture line *(arrow)* within a localized sclerotic *(white)* area at the mid to distal aspect of the medial border.

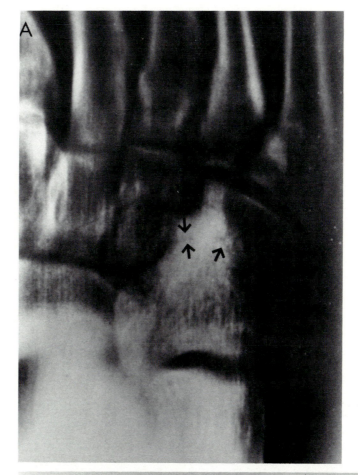

B, Radionuclide bone scan demonstrates a localized area of augmented isotope uptake at the medial border of the cuboid, best seen on the plantar (see Fig 1–27) and lateral views.

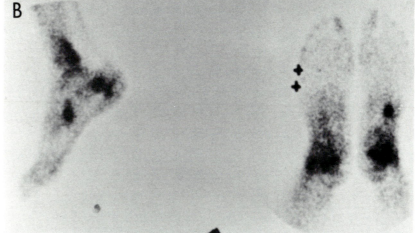

Stress Fracture—Cuboid

REMEDY   Limited activity until asymptomatic.

Avulsion Injury—Cuboid

FIG 1–38.
Avulsion fracture from the distal aspect of
the cuboid *(arrow)*.

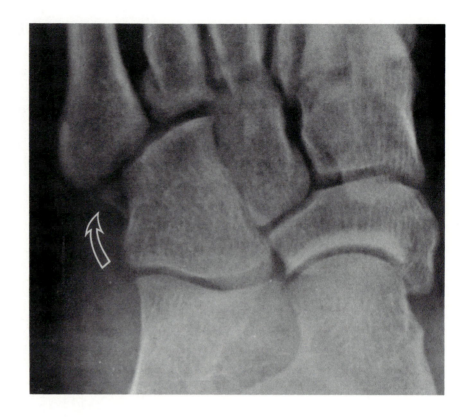

Avulsion Injury—Cuboid

REMEDY   Non-weight-bearing cast immobilization and crutches.

CALCANEUS

Juxta-articular Ossicles—Os Calcaneus Secondarius

FIG 1–39.
The os calcaneus secondarius is located at the anterior process of the calcaneus. The ossicle is well corticated with slightly beveled margins. This roentgen finding cannot be distinguished from an old injury in which the fragment has healed as an ununited fracture.

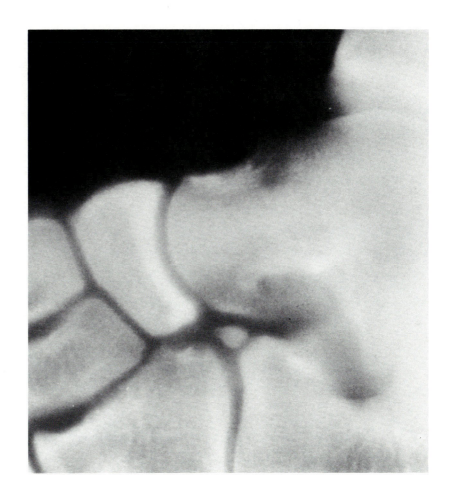

Juxta-articular Ossicles—Os Calcaneus Secondarius

REMEDY If symptomatic, surgical excision of the ununited ossicle.

Avulsion Injury—Anterior Process of Calcaneus

Avulsion injuries of the calcaneus occur at the anterior superior process secondary to the bifurcate ligament origin and at the lateral distal aspect secondary to the extensor digitorum brevis origin.

Anterior Process of Calcaneus

The bifurcate ligament originates on the anterior process of the calcaneus and inserts on the navicular and cuboid. An avulsion injury is usually the result of forefoot adduction.

FIG 1–40.

A, An acute fracture of the anterior process of calcaneus in which the fragments "fit" together. (*Continued.*)

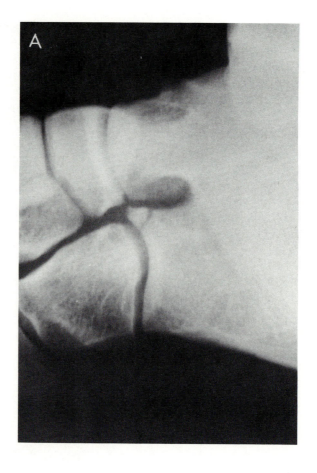

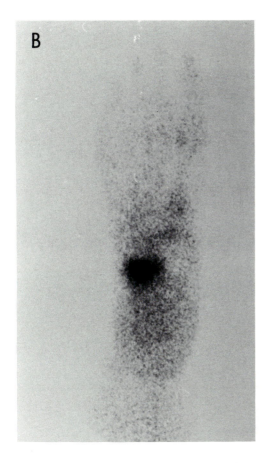

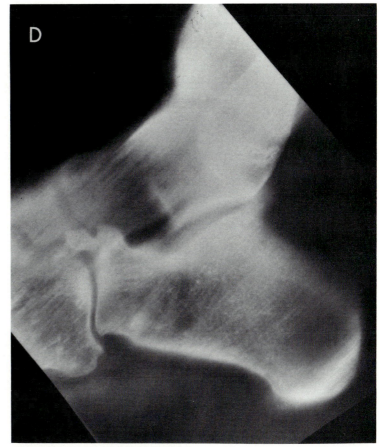

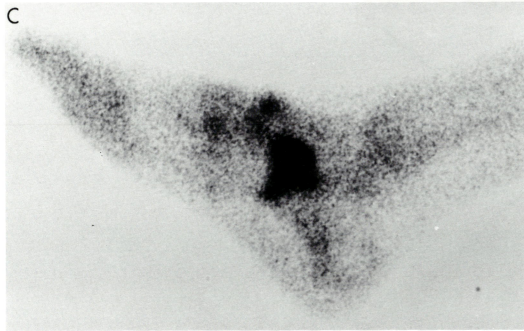

FIG 1–40 (cont.).
B, C, D (all same patient), The fracture of the anterior process of the calcaneus may be difficult to identify on a routine radiograph, but a radionuclide bone scan will demonstrate localized augmented isotope uptake, and a lateral tomogram (**D**) documents the fracture and, in this instance, a nonunion. *(Continued.)*

Avulsion Injury—Anterior Process of Calcaneus (cont.)

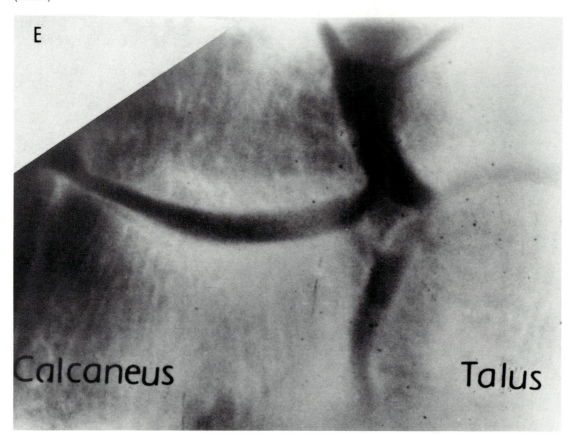

FIG 1–40 (cont.).
E, A well corticated rectangular density in the region of the anterior superior process of the calcaneus represents either an os calcaneus secondarius, old ununited fracture fragment, or post-traumatic myositis ossificans within the bifurcate ligament.

Avulsion Injury—Anterior Process of Calcaneus

REMEDY   *Acute injury:* immobilization with non-weight-bearing cast. *Non-union:* if symptomatic, surgical excision of the ununited fragment.

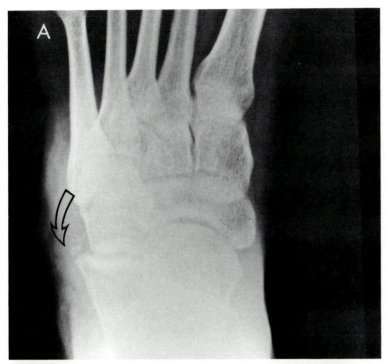

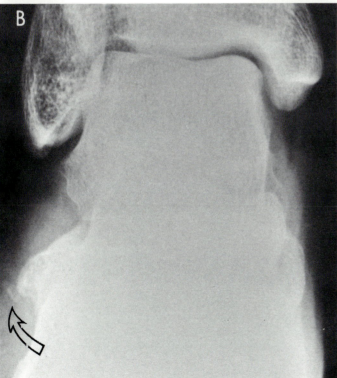

Avulsion Injury—Distal Lateral Aspect of Calcaneus

Distal Lateral Aspect of Calcaneus
The extensor digitorum brevis inserts on the lateral aspect of the calcaneus and an avulsion fracture is usually secondary to forefoot abduction. The fracture and associated soft tissue swelling are identified on the AP view of the foot and/or ankle.

FIG 1–41.
A, B (both same patient), The fracture is identified on the AP view of the foot adjacent to the distal lateral border of the calcaneus (*arrow*) (**A**) and on the AP view of the ankle adjacent to the lateral margin of the calcaneus. (*Continued.*)

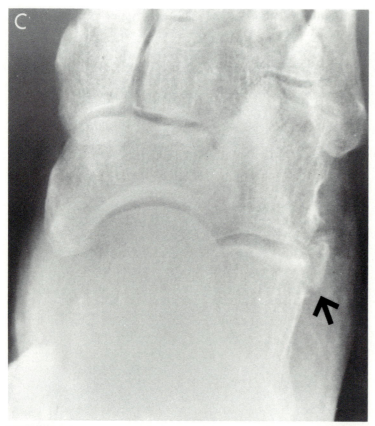

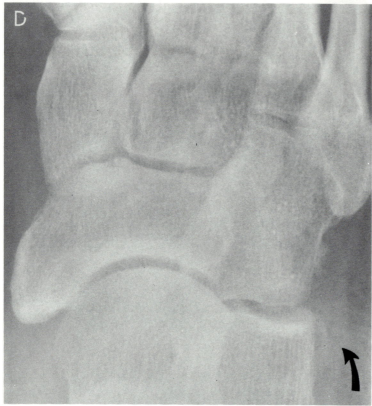

FIG 1–41 (cont.).
C, D, On the AP view of the foot, the fracture *(arrow)* is identified adjacent to the distal lateral border of the calcaneus. *(Continued.)*

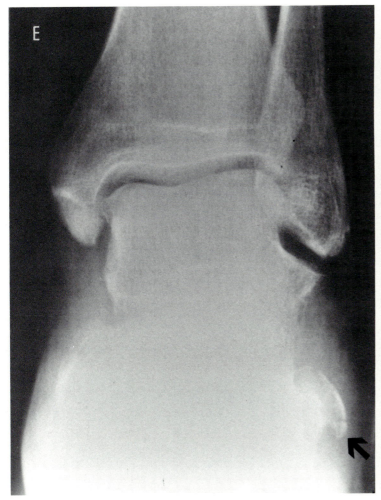

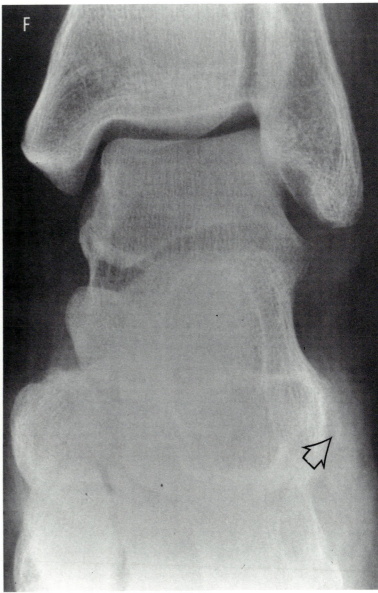

FIG 1-41 (cont.)
E (same patient as **C**), **F** (same patient as **D**), On the AP view of the ankle, the fracture *(arrow)* is identified adjacent to the lateral margin of the calcaneus. (Ref: Norfray J, Rogers LF, Adamo GP, et al: Common calcaneal avulsion fractures. *AJR* 1980; 134:119.)

Avulsion Injury—Distal Lateral Aspect of Calcaneus

REMEDY *Acute injury:* compression wrap, crutches, and non-weight-bearing.

Stress Fracture—Calcaneus

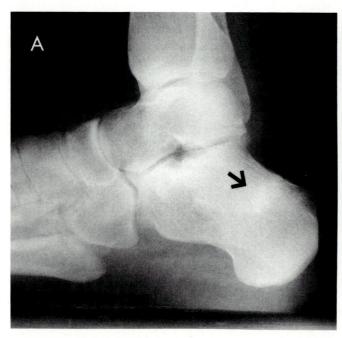

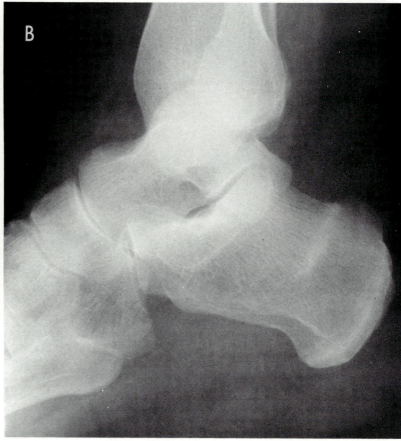

FIG 1–42.
A–C, Stress fractures are vertically oriented linear radiodensities *(arrow)* in the dorsal posterior half of the calcaneus as shown in these three patients. *(Continued).*

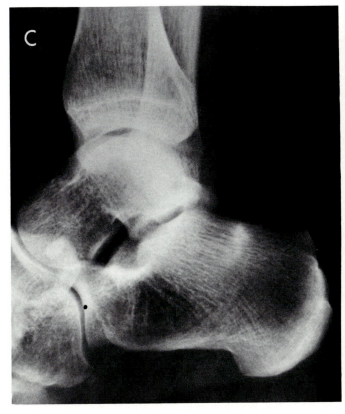

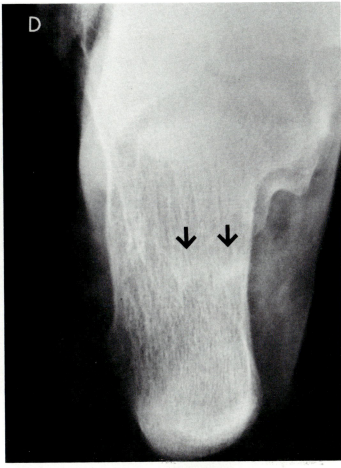

FIG 1–42 (cont.).
On the Harris view (**D,** same patient as **C**), the linear radiodensity *(arrows)* is perpendicular to the longitudinal axis of the calcaneus.

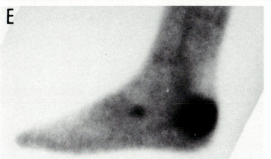

E, Radionuclide bone scan views demonstrate augmented isotope uptake in the posterior calcaneus.

Stress Fracture—Calcaneus

REMEDY   Limited activity until painfree.

Necrosis—Sever's Disease

FIG 1–43.
Lateral view of a child's foot demonstrates a
dense calcaneal apophysis. This finding is
normal and indicates that the child is walking. The retrocalcaneal recess is lucent and
normal *(arrow)*.

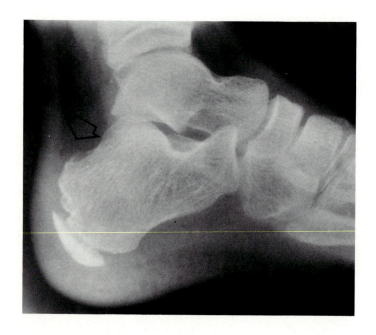

Necrosis—Sever's Disease

REMEDY   In children with a painful heel and normal roentgen findings, a
heel cup, activity modification, and reassurance of the self-lim-
ited nature of pain.

POSTERIOR HINDFOOT—SOFT TISSUE INJURIES

Normal Findings Including Parallel Pitch Lines

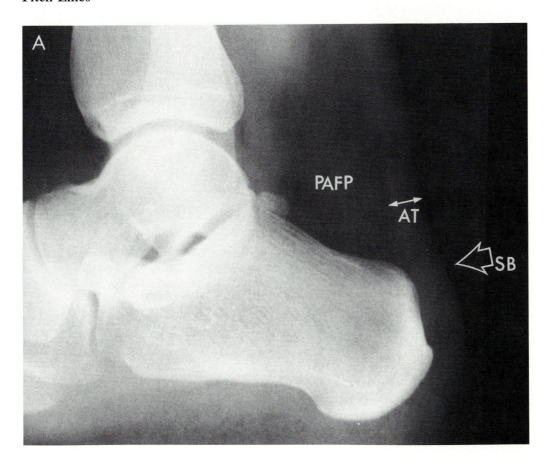

FIG 1–44.

A, The Achilles tendon *(AT)* is measured 2 cm above the bursal projection *(BP)* or the posterior superior dome of the calcaneus, and normally measures between 4 and 9 mm in the AP diameter. The anterior border of the Achilles tendon is sharply demarcated by the interface with the pre-Achilles fat pad *(PAFP)*. The superficial Achilles bursa *(SB)* is an adventitious bursa that forms in response to trauma and inflammation and the soft tissues posterior to the bursal projection are normally concave. *(Continued.)*

Normal Findings Including Parallel Pitch Lines (cont.)

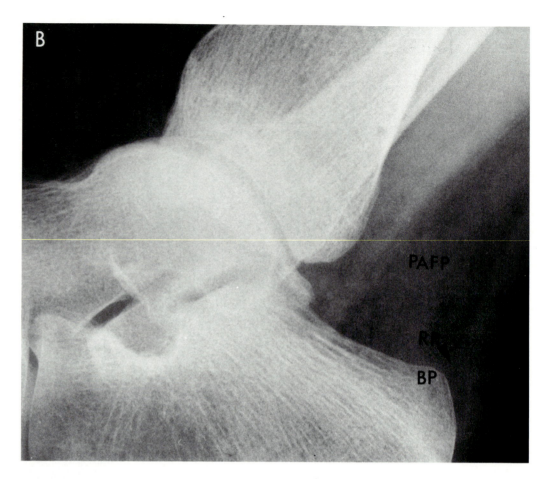

FIG 1–44 (cont.).
B, Close-up view demonstrates the normal radiolucent retrocalcaneal recess *(RR)*, located between the Achilles tendon and the bursal projection *(BP)*; it is the inferior extent of the pre-Achilles fat pad *(PAFP)*. A lucent retrocalcaneal recess indicates a normal retrocalcaneal bursa. *(Continued.)*

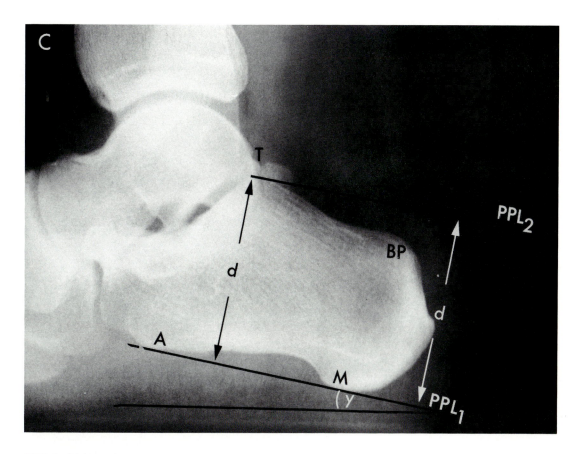

FIG 1–44 (cont.).
C, The parallel pitch lines (PPL) are constructed on a standing lateral view of the foot. The PPL$_1$ is a line drawn tangent to the anterior (A) and medial (M) tuberosities. The PPL$_2$ is constructed parallel to PPL$_1$ at the perpendicular distance (d) between PPL$_1$ and the talar articular (T). The bursal projection is considered to be normal if it falls below this PPL$_2$ and is referred to as a − PPL. The calcaneal pitch is the inclination of the heel and is determined by the angle formed by the PPL$_1$ and the horizontal (angle y). Note that the medial tuberosity is not large. (Permission for **B, C** granted courtesy of Pavlov H, Heneghan M, Hersh A, et al: The Haglund syndrome: Initial and differential diagnosis. *Radiology* 1982; 144:83.)

Isolated Superficial Tendo Achilles Bursitis

FIG 1–45.
There is a localized soft tissue bulge *(arrows)* or convexity posterior to the calcaneal bursal projection. The retrocalcaneal recess and Achilles tendon are normal.

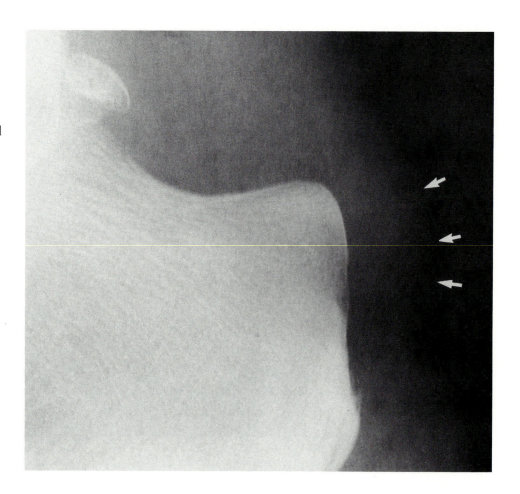

Isolated Superficial Tendo Achilles Bursitis

REMEDY　　　　　Shoe modification with heel left and steroid/xylocaine injection into bursa.

Isolated Retrocalcaneal Bursitis

FIG 1–46.
Retrocalcaneal bursitis is diagnosed by loss of the radiolucent retrocalcaneal recess *(arrow).* The Achilles tendon is clearly delineated.

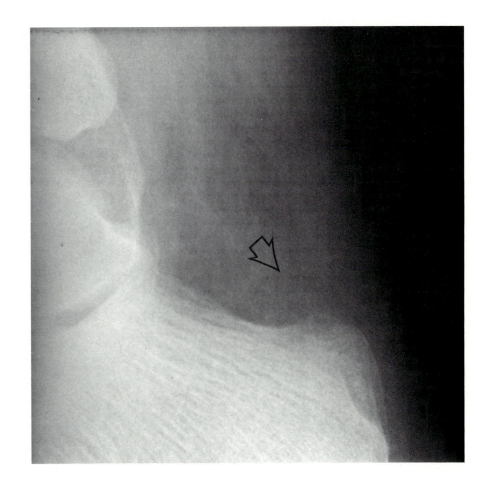

Isolated Retrocalcaneal Bursitis

REMEDY   Shoe modification with heel lift and steroid/xylocaine injection into bursa.

Haglund's Disease

FIG 1–47

A, B (both same patient), Clinically, there is a "pump bump," i.e., thickening and prominence of the Achilles tendon insertion as demonstrated in this patient (*arrows*) (left heel). (*Continued.*)

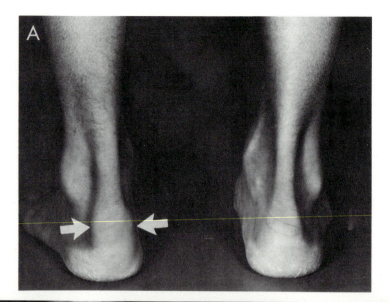

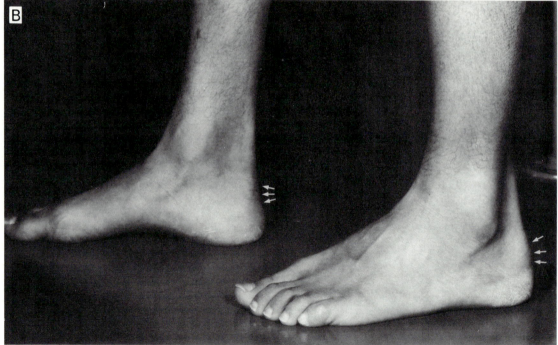

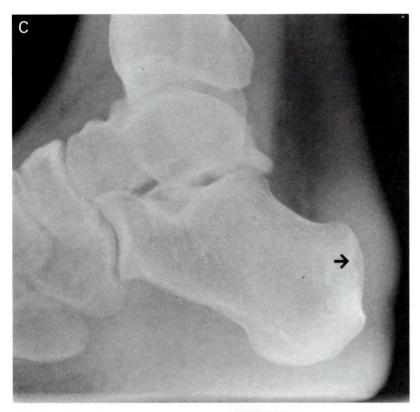

FIG 1–47 (cont.).
C–F, Radiographically, Haglund's disease presents with the following findings: (1) Achilles tendinitis, thickening of the Achilles tendon, and loss of delineation between the Achilles tendon and the pre-Achilles fat pad; (2) retrocalcaneal bursitis, loss of the radiolucent retrocalcaneal recess; (3) superficial tendo Achilles bursitis, swelling and convexity posterior to the Achilles tendon insertion; and (4) a +PPL. Occasionally, a subchondral cyst is present in the calcaneus *(arrow)* (**C**), or calcification at the insertion site of the Achilles tendon (**D**). *(Continued.)*

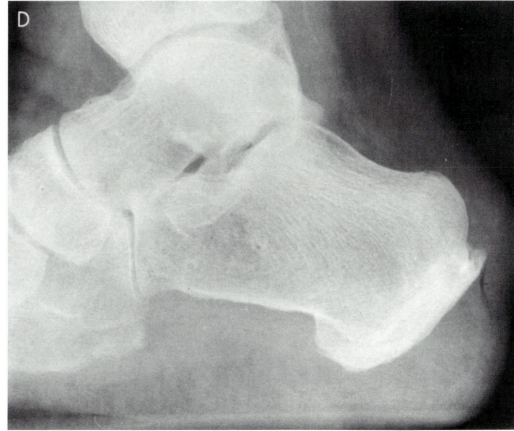

Haglund's Disease (cont.)

FIG 1–47 (cont.).
E, F, Parallel pitch lines demonstrate a prominent bursal projection, a +*PPL* (i.e., the bursal projection (*BP*) extends beyond the top PPL_2.) Compare to normal in Fig 1–44, C. The calcaneal pitch is steep secondary to a large medial tuberosity (*M*) referred to as a plantar osseous projection. A large plantar osseous projection increases the calcaneus pitch and the effective prominence of the bursal projection. (*Continued.*)

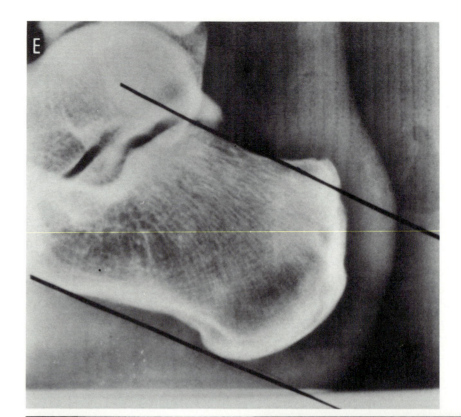

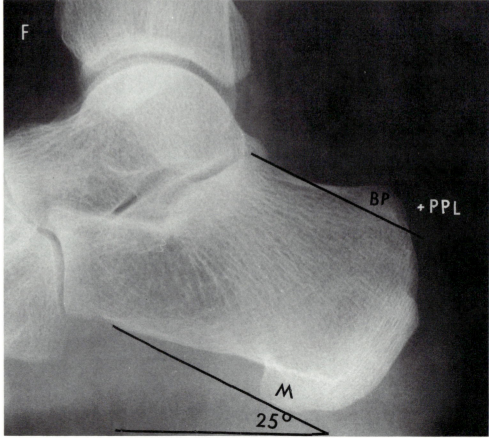

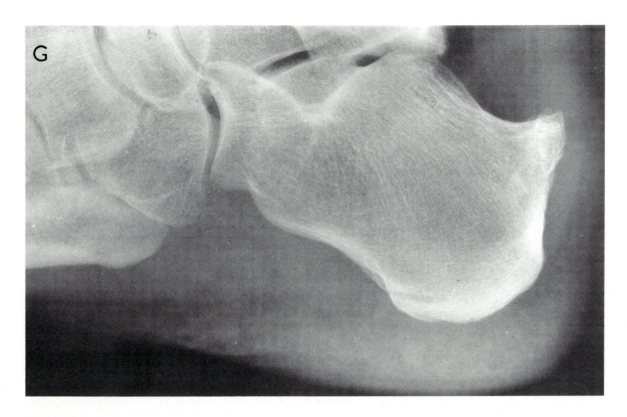

FIG 1–47 (cont.).
G, Lateral view of the calcaneus demonstrates an extremely prominent and jagged bursal projection, a retrocalcaneal exostosis. The clinically evident "pump bump" is formed by the normal soft tissues being pushed posteriorly by the prominent bursal projection. (Permission for **A, B, D, G** granted courtesy of Pavlov H, Heneghan M, Hersh A, et al: The Haglund syndrome: Initial and differential diagnosis. *Radiology* 1982; 144:83.)

Haglund's Disease

REMEDY   Shoe modification, heel lift, steroid injection. If symptoms are unresponsive to conservative measures, excision of the bursal projection. An example of surgery is demonstrated by Figures **a, b. a,** Initial films demonstrate the planned surgical removal of a prominent bursal projection in a patient with Haglund's disease. **b,** Immediate postoperative films demonstrate the calcaneus after the prominent bursal projection was removed.

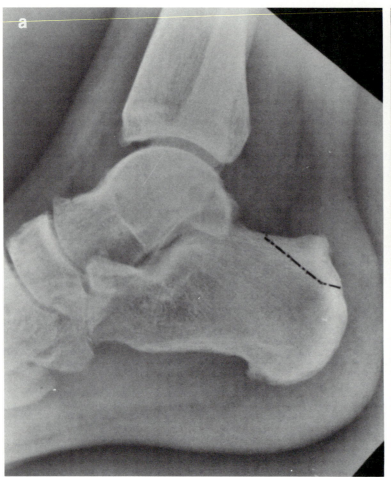
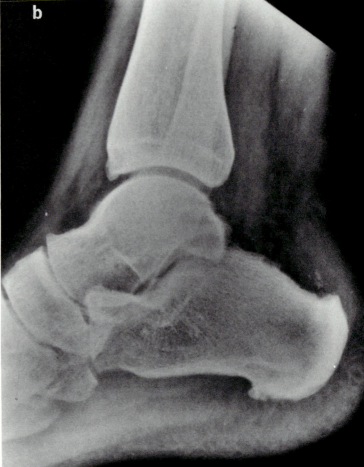

Systemic Disease

FIG 1–48.
Lateral view of the foot demonstrates all the findings of Haglund's disease; i.e., a "pump bump" with increase in the radiographic density of the soft tissues posterior to the bursal projection, a retrocalcaneal bursitis with loss of the radiolucent retrocalcaneal recess, and Achilles tendinitis with increase in the width of the Achilles tendon and loss of the definition between the Achilles tendon and pre-Achilles fat pad; however, there are erosions on the posterior cortex of the calcaneus. Cortical erosions are suggestive of a systemic inflammatory process such as Reiter's syndrome or rheumatoid arthritis. (Permission granted courtesy of Pavlov H, Heneghan M, Hersh A, et al: The Haglund syndrome: Initial and differential diagnosis. *Radiology* 1982; 144:83.)

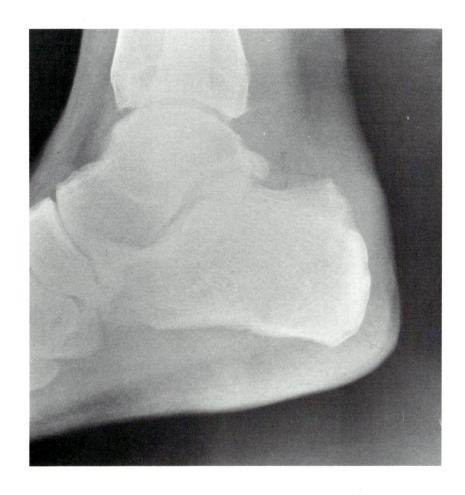

Systemic Disease

REMEDY   Local treatment as for Haglund's disease with a medical evaluation for possible systemic disease.

Calcific Achilles Tendinitis

FIG 1–49.
A, Calcification within the Achilles tendon and a poorly defined tendon indicates calcific tendinitis. *(Continued).*

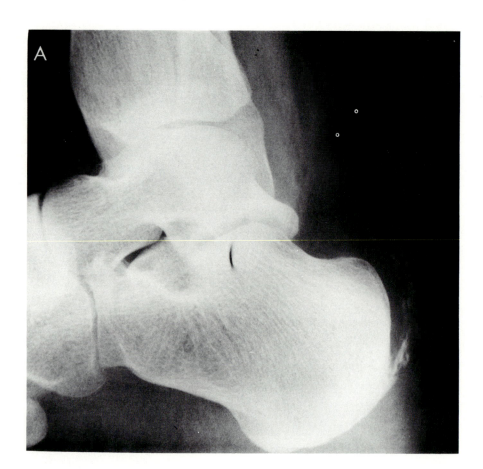

FIG 1–49 (cont.).
B, Well-defined calcifications at the insertion site of the Achilles tendon *(arrows)* are usually of no clinical significance. The retrocalcaneal recess *(arrowhead)* and the Achilles tendon are normal.

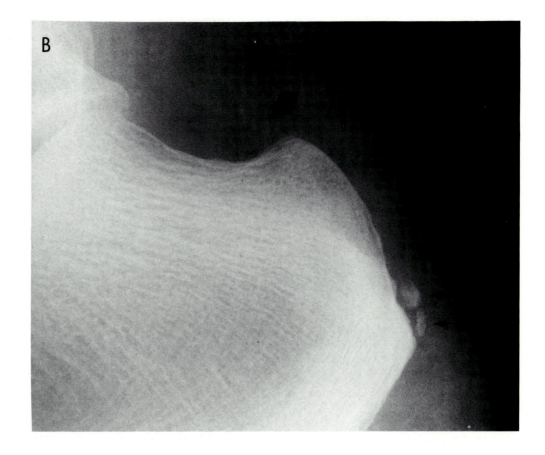

Calcific Achilles Tendinitis

REMEDY   Ice, anti-inflammatory drug, stretching exercises, and corrective orthotics with round flared heel and sturdy heel counter. If the patient has a +PPL, the bursal projection should be excised.

Achilles Tendon Rupture

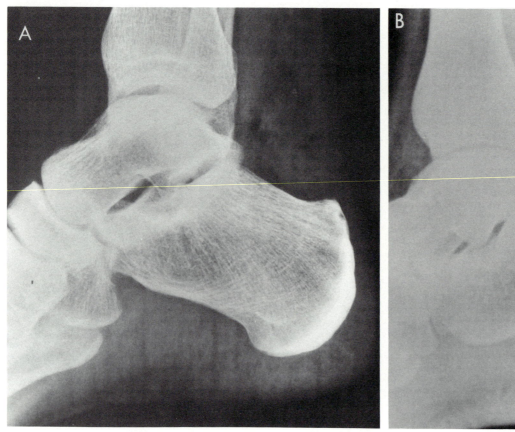 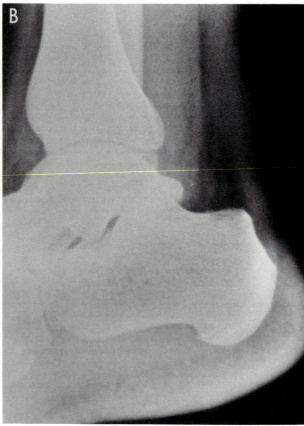

FIG 1–50.
A, The Achilles tendon shadow is not present. The black streaks of air within the regional soft tissues indicate an open laceration of the tendon.

B, Lateral view demonstrates localized thickening of the Achilles tendon approximately 4 cm above the top of the calcaneus. In the appropriate clinical setting, this finding is consistent with an acute rupture of the Achilles tendon. *(Continued.)*

FIG 1–50 (cont.).
C, The Achilles tendon has a fusiform contour *(arrows)*. The delineation between the anterior edge of the Achilles tendon and the pre-Achilles fat pad is poorly defined, and the AP dimension of the Achilles tendon is over 9 mm (measured 2 cm above the calcaneus) indicating a partial intersubstance tear. The age of the tear is indeterminate. *(Continued.)*

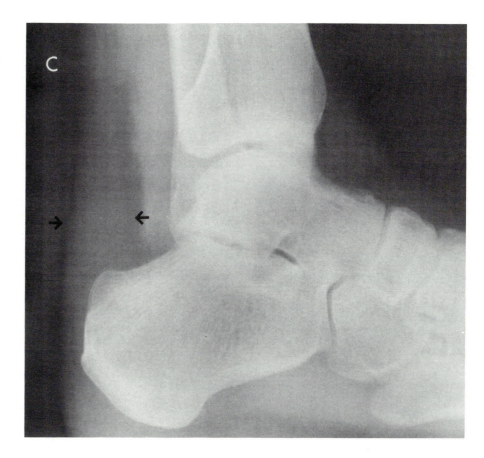

ACHILLES TENDON RUPTURE
(cont.)

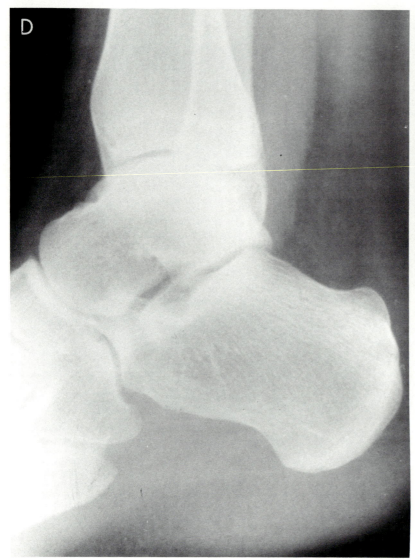

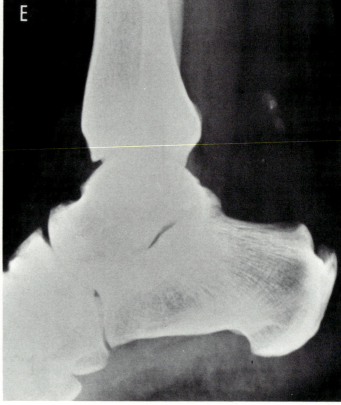

FIG 1–50 (cont.).
D, The major portion of the Achilles tendon shadow is absent although the insertion of the Achilles tendon appears normal indicating a complete tear of the tendon. The age of the tear is indeterminate.

E, Calcification within the substance of the tendon, and a poorly delineated tendon indicates a healed tendon injury.

Achilles Tendon Rupture

REMEDY   *Partial intersubstance tear:* stretching exercises but surgical decompression and debridement if unresponsive to conservative management. *Complete rupture:* surgical reapproximation.

Accessory Muscles of the Lower Calf

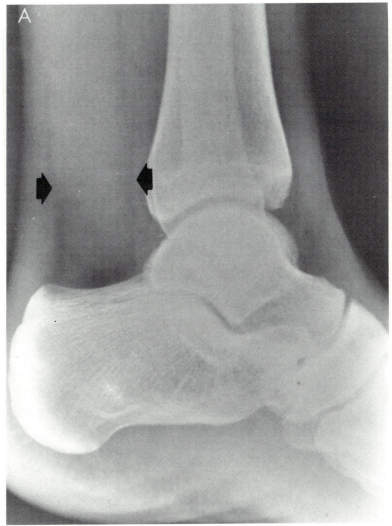

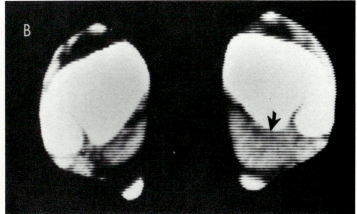

FIG 1–51.
A, B (both same patient), The density (between *arrows*) within the pre-Achilles fat pad represents an accessory muscle covering the posterior tibial neurovascular bundle.

B, On CT, this is seen as an enlarged muscle mass *(arrow)* in the pre-Achilles fat pad anterior to the Achilles tendon. This accessory muscle is of no clinical significance. (Ref: Nidecker AC, Von Hochstetter A, Fredenhagen H: Accessory muscles of the lower calf. *Radiology* 1984; 151:47–48.)

Accessory Muscles of the Lower Calf

REMEDY   None.

Plantar Fasciitis

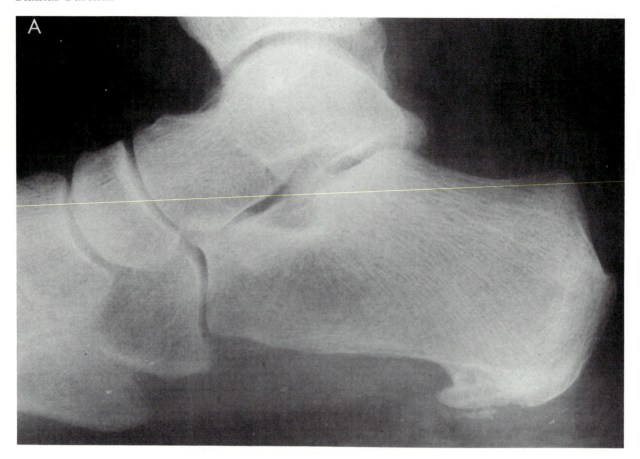

FIG 1–52.
A, There is calcification within the plantar fascia, inferior to a large calcaneal spur. (Permission granted courtesy of Pavlov H, Torg JS, Hersh A, et al: The roentgen examination of runners' injuries. *Radio-Graphics* 1981; 1:17–34.) *(Continued.)*

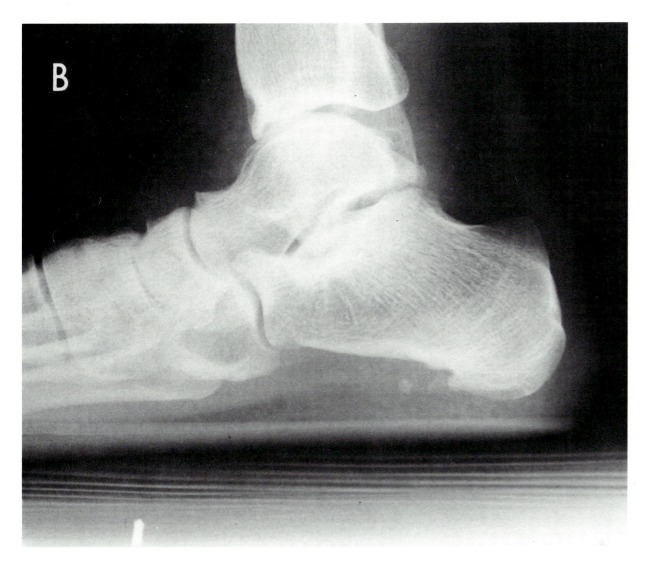

FIG 1–52 (cont.).
B, Calcification within the plantar fascia anterior to a calcaneal spur.

Plantar Fasciitis (cont.)

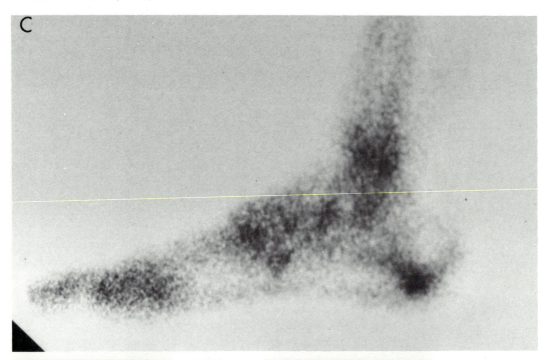

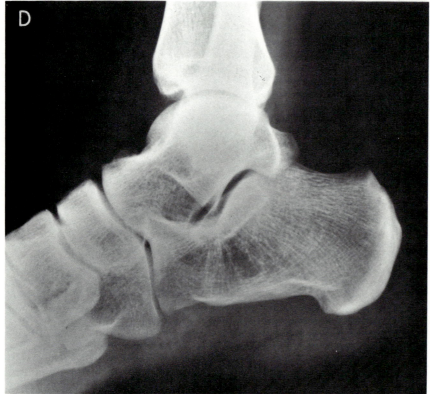

C, D (both same patient) Plantar fasciitis can be diagnosed by a radionuclide bone scan by localized augmented isotope uptake when there is insufficient calcification to be detected radiographically (**D**).

Plantar Fasciitis

REMEDY

Low Dye strapping, heel cup, felt "donut," arch support, steroid injection, and stretching exercises. Occasionally, surgical release of plantar fascia is required. In addition to plantar fascial release, heel spur excision may be indicated, as demonstrated on preoperative **(a)** and postoperative **(b)** radiographs.

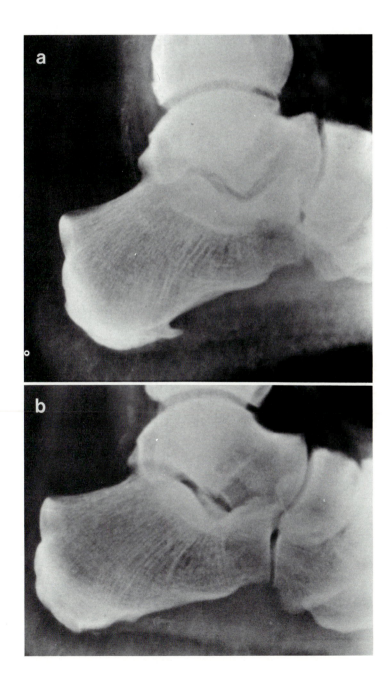

CHAPTER 2

The Ankle

TIBIAL-TALAR JOINT

Hypertrophic Talar and Tibial Proliferative Osteophytes

FIG 2–1.
A, Hypertrophic spur on the dorsal surface of the talus occurs secondary to micro-trauma at the ankle capsule insertion and may abut against the anterior tibial lip in dorsiflexion.

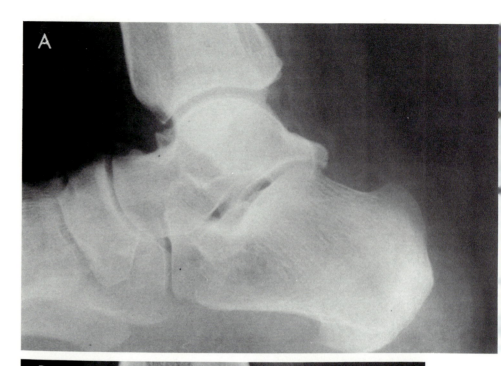

B, Hypertrophic proliferative changes from the anterior tibial lip producing painful dorsiflexion. Note associated soft-tissue swelling and inflammation. *(Continued.)*

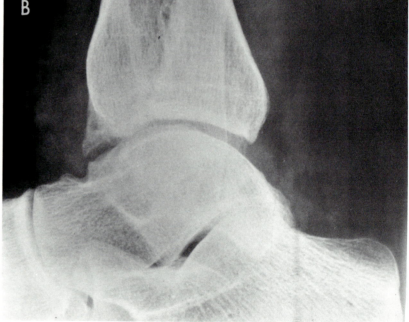

FIG 2–1 (cont.)
C, Hypertrophic proliferative spurs projecting from both the talus and anterior tibial
lip.

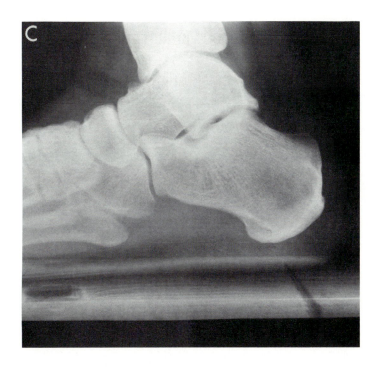

Hypertrophic Talar and Tibial Proliferative Osteophytes

REMEDY   Excision of symptomatic proliferative spur.

Fracture of Hypertrophic Tibial Osteophyte

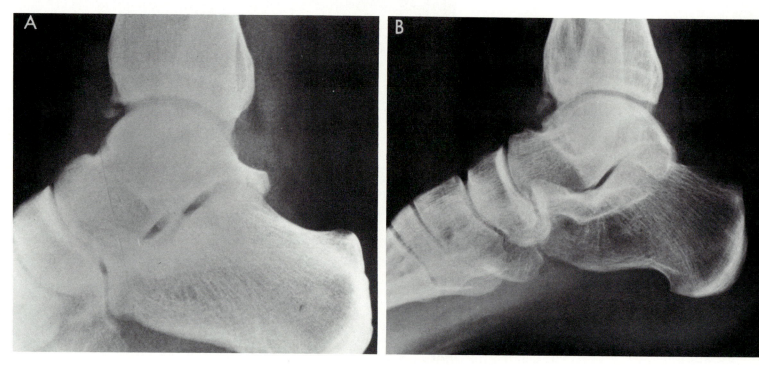

FIG 2–2.
A, B, Fractures of the anterior tibial osteophytic spur.

Fracture of Hypertrophic Tibial Osteophyte

REMEDY   If significant symptomatology due to a fibrous union, surgical removal of fracture fragment is indicated.

TALUS

Osteochondritis Dissecans—Talus

FIG 2–3.
A, B (both same patient), Radiolucency at the superior medial dome of the talus (*arrow*) representing post-traumatic osteochondritis dissecans.

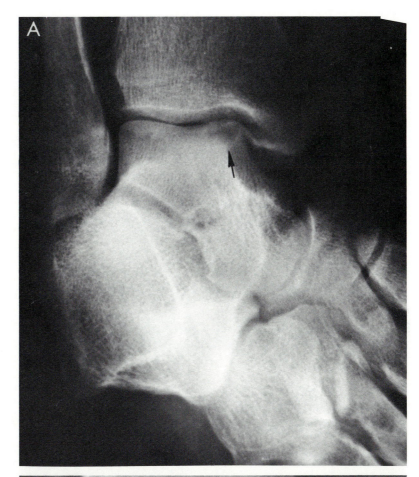

B, A tomogram performed following a double contrast arthrogram demonstrates an intact articular cartilage (*arrowhead*) overlying the radiolucent osseous defect (*arrow*). (Permission for **A, B** granted courtesy of Pavlov H: Ankle and subtalar arthrography. In Symposium of Ankle and Foot Problems in the Athlete. *Clin Sports Med* 1982; 1:47–69.) (*Continued.*)

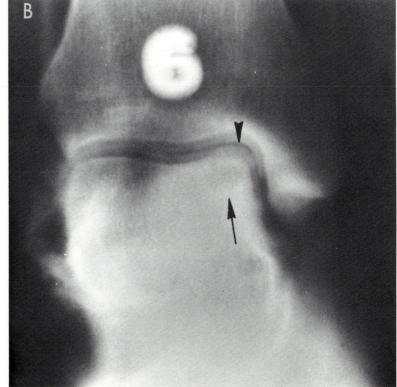

Osteochondritis Dissecans—Talus (cont.)

FIG 2–3 (cont.).
C, D (both same patient), A sclerotic osseous body is present within the radiolucent post-traumatic osteochondritis dissecans at the medial talar dome.

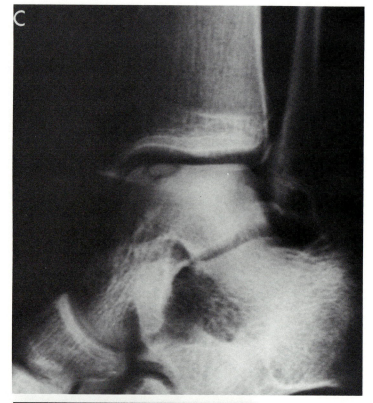

D, An axial computed tomography (CT) image through the talar dome demonstrates the separate osseous body *(arrow)*. *(Continued.)*

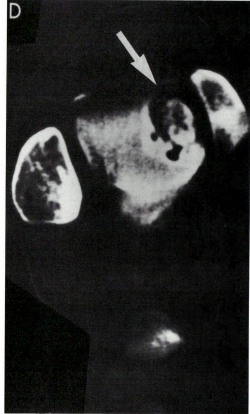

FIG 2–3 (cont.).
E, F (both same patient), There is a notch defect *(arrow)* in the superior medial dome of the talus.

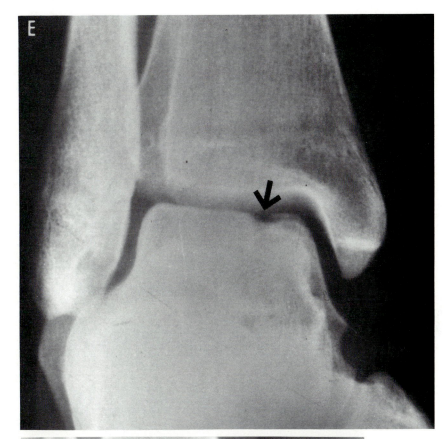

F, An arthrotomogram demonstrates the articular cartilage over the osseous notch defect to be intact *(Continued.)*

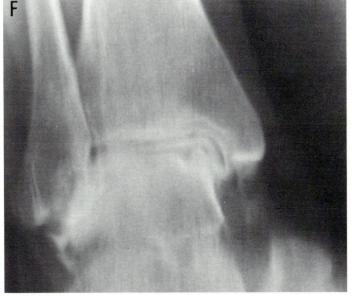

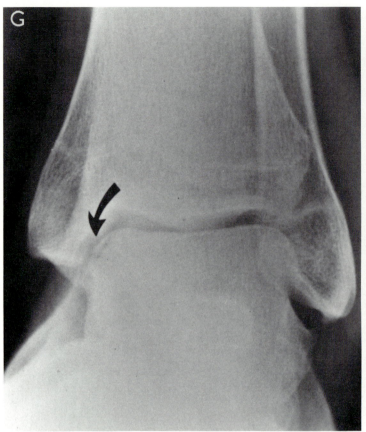

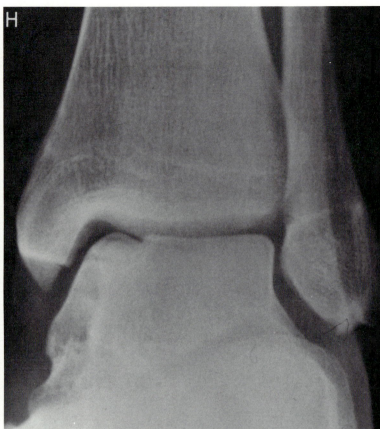

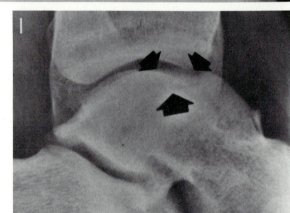

Osteochondritis Dissecans—Talus (cont.)

FIG 2–3 (cont.).
G–I (all same patient), On the anteroposterior (AP) view (**G**) and mortise view (**H**), a subchondral lucent defect is present at the medial dome of talar articular surface (*arrow*).

I, A large circular osseous body is seen on the lateral view (*arrows*).

Osteochondritis Dissecans—Talus

REMEDY   *In adolescents:* a symptomatic osteochondritis dissecans is treated with a non-weight-bearing short leg cast and immobilization for 6–8 weeks. *In adults or adolescents with persistent pain and swelling:* surgery is recommended.

Transchondral and Osteochondral Fracture

FIG 2–4.
A, There is a nondisplaced osteochondral fracture fragment at the lateral dome of the talus *(arrow)*.

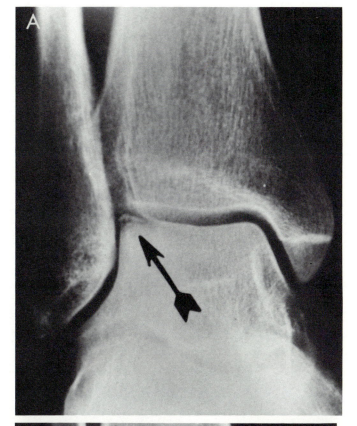

B, An arthrogram demonstrates a loose chondral fragment *(arrows)* at the superior medial dome of the talus. (Permission for **A, B** granted courtesy of Pavlov H: Ankle and subtalar arthrography. In Symposium of Ankle and Foot Problems in the Athlete. *Clin Sports Med* 1982; 1:47–69.)

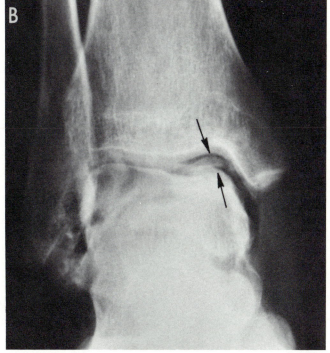

Transchondral and Osteochondral Fracture

REMEDY   Excision of osteochondral fragment.

INTRA-ARTICULAR

Joint Effusion

FIG 2–5.
A, B, Lateral view demonstrates soft-tissue density anterior to tibial talar joint *(arrows)* indicating an effusion.

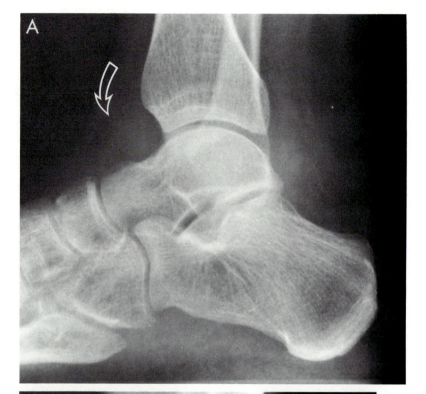

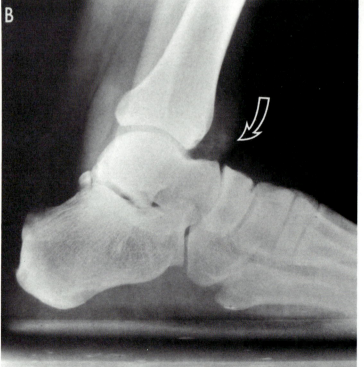

Joint Effusion—Intra-articular

REMEDY   Determine etiology of effusion. This may require clinical, roentgenographic, arthrographic, and/or arthroscopic examination and/or fluid analysis.

Loose Bodies

FIG 2–6.
A, Lateral view demonstrates a small osseous body *(arrows)* in the ankle mortise.
Malalignment of the tibial talar articular
surfaces indicates ligmentous instability.

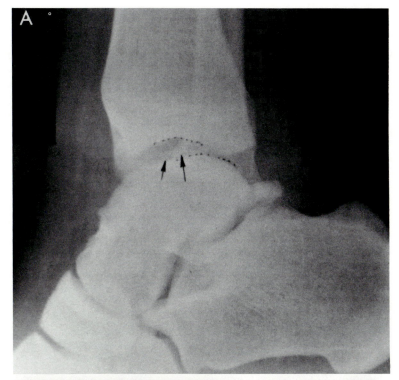

B, Lateral view following a single contrast
arthrogram demonstrates intra-articular
loose bodies in the anterior and posterior
compartments of the ankle joint *(arrows).*
(Permission for **B** granted courtesy of Pavlov H: Ankle and subtalar Arthrography. In
Symposium of Ankle and Foot Problems in
the Athlete. *Clin Sports Med* 1982;
1:47–69.)

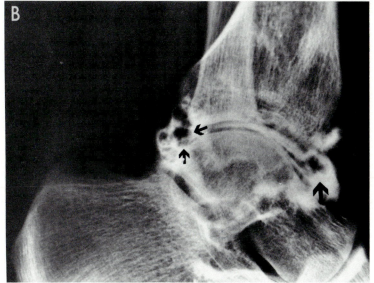

Loose Bodies—Intra-articular

REMEDY   Arthrotomy: removal of loose bodies and repair of disrupted ligaments.

NONOSSEOUS INJURIES

Ligamentous Injuries and Ankle Instability

Routine Radiographs

FIG 2–7.
A, A lateral view obtained with anterior stress on the foot demonstrates anterior subluxation of the talus with respect to the tibia. A positive anterior drawer sign indicates a rupture of the anterior talofibular and the fibular calcaneal ligament.

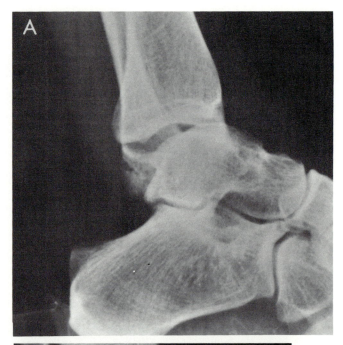

B, Inversion stress view demonstrates widening of the lateral aspect of the ankle mortise. Comparison examination with the contralateral side must be used as a standard to determine the degree of post-traumatic, as opposed to physiologic, laxity. *(Continued.)*

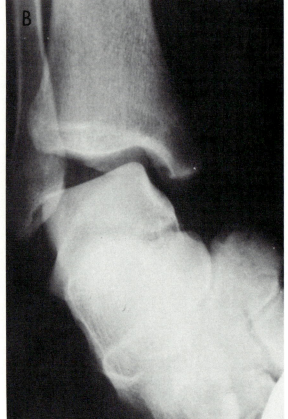

Arthrograms

FIG 2–7 (cont.).
C, D (both same patient), Following an arthrogram, contrast is noted surrounding the distal fibula indicating an acute tear of the anterior talofibular ligament.

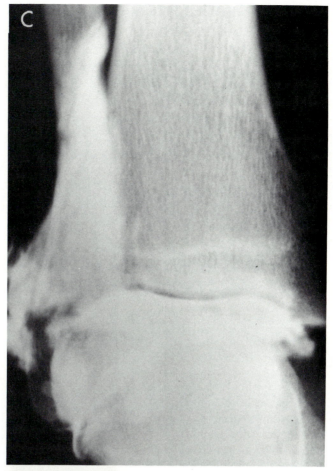

D, During inversion stress, there is widening of the lateral aspect of the ankle mortise. *(Continued.)*

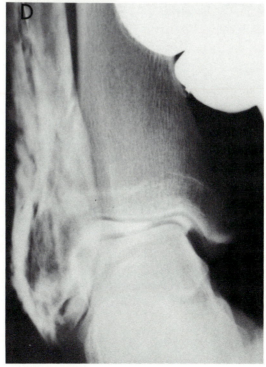

Ligamentous Injuries and Ankle Instability (cont.)

FIG 2–7 (cont.).

E, Contrast lateral to the fibula indicates an acute anterior talofibular ligament tear. The contrast between the tibia and fibula extending proximally over 2.5 cm from the ankle mortise indicates a diastasis of the interosseous membrane. Note that the talus is displaced laterally in the mortise.

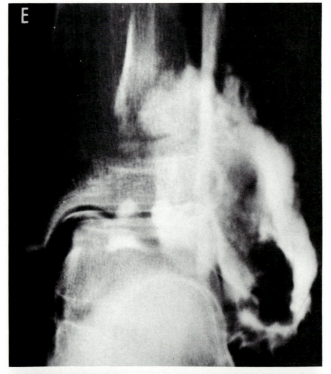

F, Rupture of the anterior talofibular and calcaneofibular ligaments. Contrast in the lateral peroneal tendon sheath *(arrows)* indicates communication with the ankle joint and represents an acute or previous calcaneofibular ligament injury. The contrast surrounding the distal fibula indicates a tear of the anterior talofibular ligament and confirms that the injury is acute. *(Continued.)*

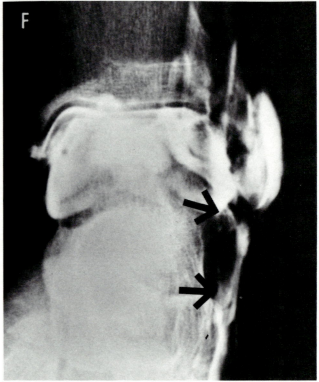

G, Contrast within the medial flexor tendon sheaths is normal. (Permission for **B, E, G** granted courtesy of Pavlov H: Ankle and subtalar Arthrography. In Symposium of Ankle and Foot Problems in the Athlete. *Clin Sports Med* 1982; 1:47–69.)

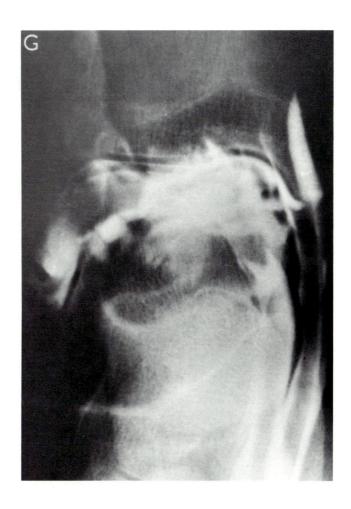

Ligamentous Injuries and Ankle Instability

REMEDY

Guidelines for management of the unstable ankle are, at best, controversial. We believe that these lesions should be divided into acute and chronic categories.

Acute Injury

One-plane instability, i.e., varus or anterior: conservative treatment with adhesive strapping, splint, or plaster immobilization.

Two-plane instability, i.e., a positive anterior draw sign associated with a positive talar tilt, varus laxity: plaster immobilization for 3 weeks; however, depending on the age and anticipated demands of the athlete, surgical repair of the involved ligaments should be considered.

Two-plane instability with involvement of the deltoid ligament: surgical repair is indicated.

Chronic Instability

One-plane instability: aggressive rehabilitated exercises particularly emphasizing dorsiflexion with utilization of the commercially available air splint.

Two-plane instability associated with recurrent injury and/or effusion: surgical reconstruction should be considered.

Chronic Interosseous Membrane Injury

FIG 2–8.
A, B, Ossification in the interosseous membrane is secondary to an old rupture. This ossification can bridge or attempt to bridge the tibia and fibula. (Permission for **B** granted courtesy of Pavlov H, Torg JS, Hersh A, et al: The roentgen examination of runners' injuries. *RadioGraphics* 1981; 1:17–34.) *(continued.)*

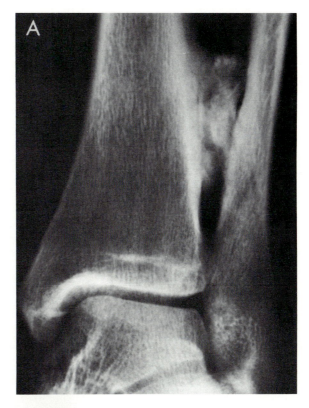

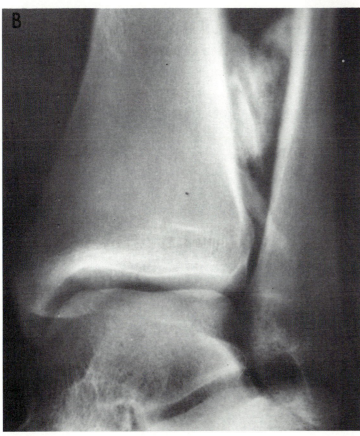

Chronic Interosseous Membrane Injury (cont.)

FIG 2–8 (cont.).
C, Ossification of interosseous membrane projects from lateral aspect of tibia and attempts to bridge both bones.

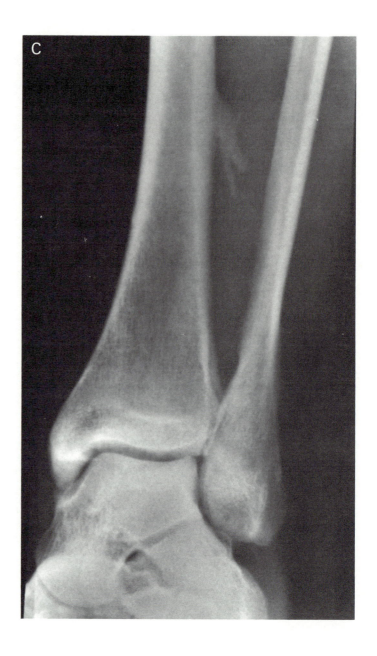

Chronic Interosseous Membrane Injury

REMEDY *Positive bone scan:* conservative treatment. *Negative bone scan:* remove cross union if symptoms are disabling.

Adhesive Capsulitis

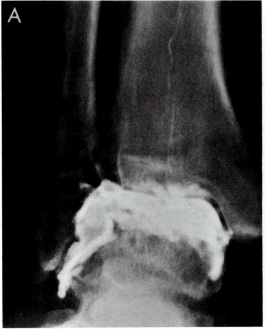

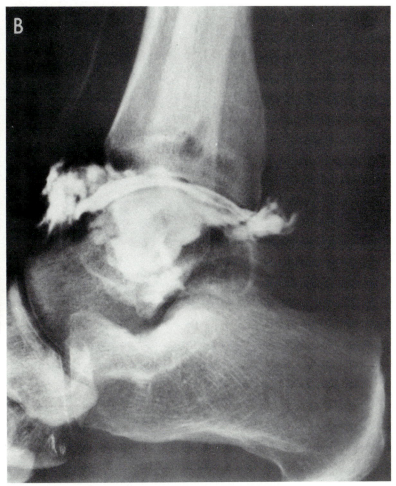

FIG 2–9.
A, B (both same patient), The synovium has a corrugated appearance and there is lymphatic uptake of contrast. This arthrographic appearance indicates an inflammatory adhesive capsulitis. (Ref: Goldman AB, Katz MC, Freiberger RH: Posttraumatic adhesive capsulitis of the ankle: Arthrographic diagnosis. *AJR* 1976; 127:585–588.) (Permission for **A, B** granted courtesy of Pavlov H: Ankle and subtalar arthrography. In Symposium of Ankle and Foot Problems in the Athlete. *Clin Sports Med* 1982; 1:47–69.)

Adhesive Capsulitis

REMEDY   Range of motion exercises and intra-articular steroid injection.

TIBIA

Stress Reaction and/or Fracture—Tibia

Nondisplaced Fracture

FIG 2–10.
Nondisplaced fracture through the intra-articular aspect of the medial tibial plafond, just at the base of the medial malleolus (*arrow*).

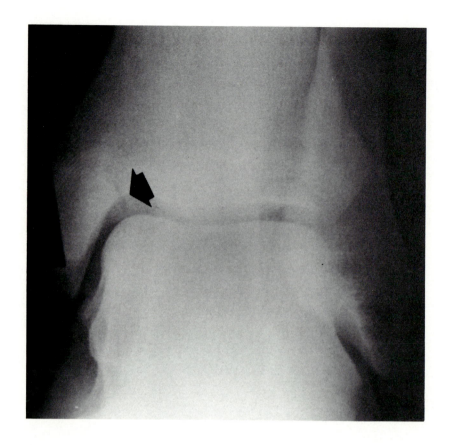

Stress Reaction and/or Fracture
Nondisplaced Fracture—Tibia

REMEDY   Non-weight-bearing cast immobilization for 6 weeks or until healed.

Cancellous Fracture

The distal tibia is cancellous bone and the typical appearance of a stress fracture in cancellous bone is a horizontal linear radiodensity.

FIG 2–11.

A–E, Three examples of cancellous stress fractures that occur just proximal to the tibial plafond. (Note: **D** and **E** appear on next page.) (Note: **B, C** same patient; **D, E** same patient.) (Permission for **D** granted courtesy of Pavlov H, Torg JS, Hersh A, et al: The roentgen examination of runners' injuries. *RadioGraphics* 1981; 1:17–34.) *(Continued.)*

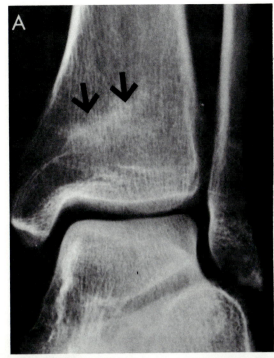

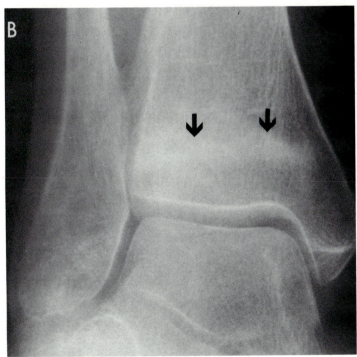

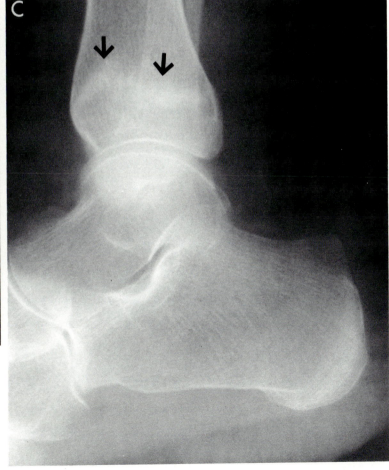

Stress Reaction and/or Fracture—Tibia (cont.)

Fig 2–11 (cont.).

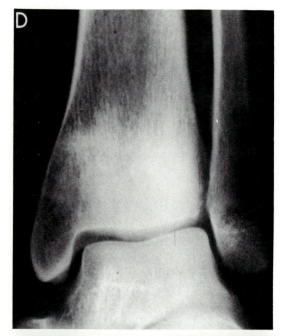

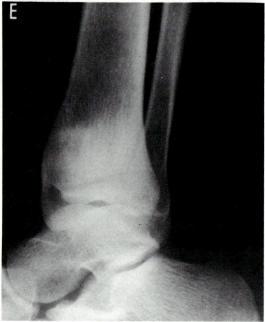

Cancellous Fracture
Stress Reaction and/or Fracture—Tibia

REMEDY   Activity limitation, orthopedic/biomechanical evaluation, and assessment of training and running habits.

CHAPTER 3

The Leg (Tibia and Fibula)

TIBIA

Stress Reaction and/or Fracture—Typical

A localized periosteal reaction and cortical thickening indicates a stress reaction or a healed stress fracture. A radiolucent line within an area of cortical thickening indicates a stress fracture. The demonstration of the fracture line is not always present on the anteroposterior (AP) and lateral views; therefore, oblique views and coned views may be required. Localized augmented isotope uptake on a radionuclide bone scan is present with either a stress reaction or a stress fracture. The typical locations for a stress reaction or a stress fracture are the posterior tibial cortex, at the junction of the middle and distal third or at the junction of the middle and proximal third.

Junction of Middle and Distal Third

FIG 3–1.
A–C (all same patient), There is a localized area of cortical hyperostosis at the medial posterior aspect of the distal tibia *(arrow)*. A definitive fracture radiolucency is not identified.
C, A radionuclide bone scan, lateral view, confirms localized augmented isotope uptake, confined to the site of posterior cortical reaction. *(Continued.)*

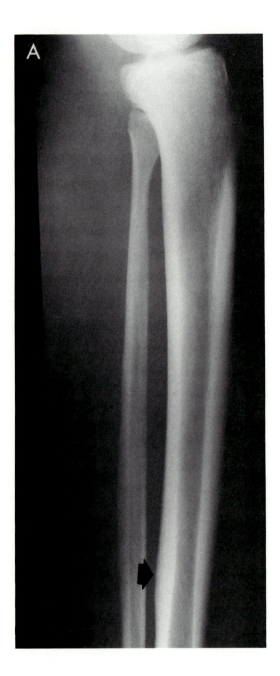

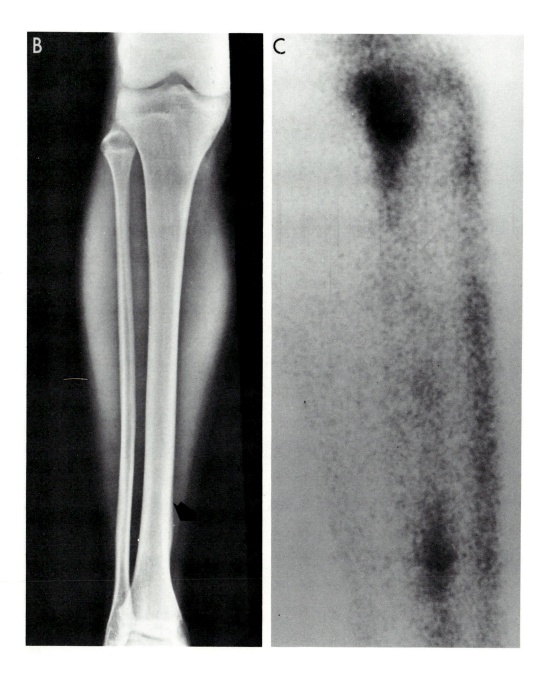

Stress Reaction and/or Fracture—Typical (cont.)

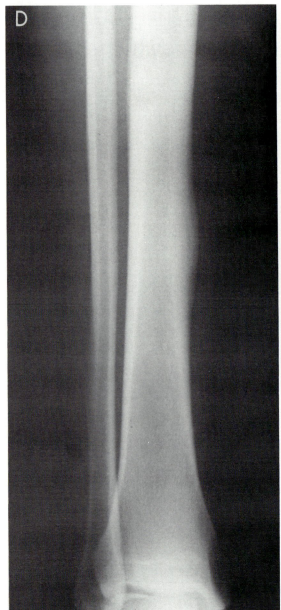

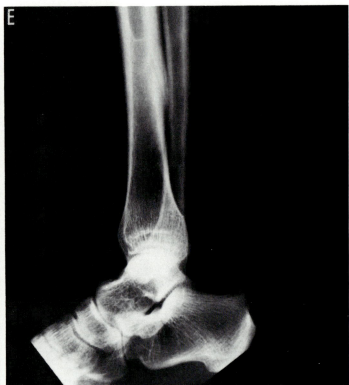

FIG 3–1 (cont.).
D, There is localized thickening of the medial cortex of the distal tibia, indicating a stress reaction or healed stress fracture; a definitive radiolucent fracture line is not evident.
E, There is an oblique radiolucent fracture line within a localized area of posterior cortical thickening. (*Continued.*)

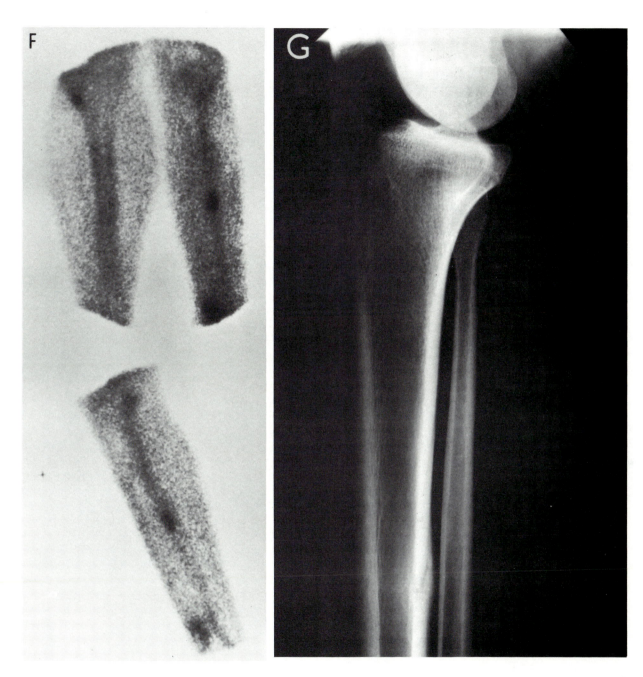

FIG 3–1 (cont.).
F, G (both same patient) Radionuclide bone scan demonstrates intense augmented isotope uptake of the midshaft of the left tibia confined to the posterior cortex.

G, Radiograph demonstrates an oblique radiolucent fracture line within the area of posterior cortical thickening. The endosteal and periosteal surfaces are both irregular. *(Continued.)*

Stress Reaction and/or Fracture—Typical (cont.)

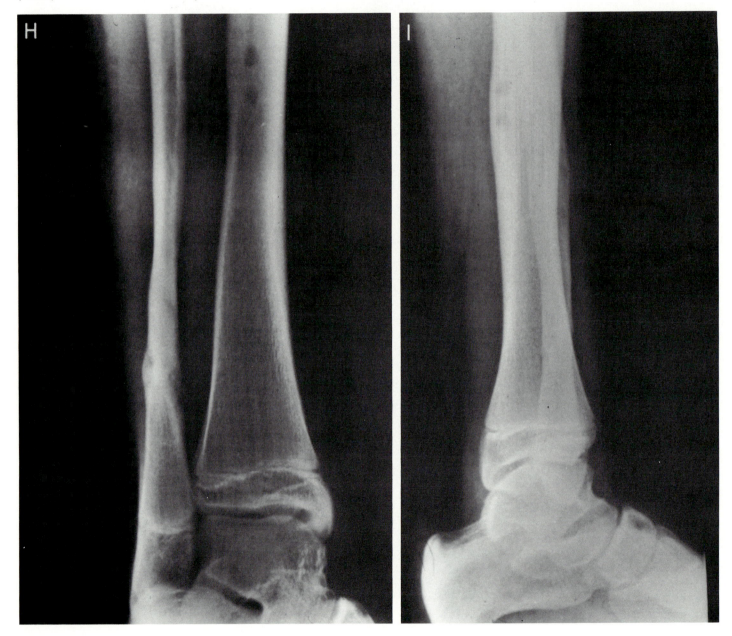

FIG 3–1 (cont.).
H, I (both same patient), On frontal and lateral views there are two circular lucencies continued within the localized thickening of the posterior tibial cortex representing residual cysts at prior stress fracture sites. There is also a healing stress fracture of the distal fibula.

Stress Reaction and/or Fracture—Typical

Junction of the Middle and Distal Third

REMEDY   Activity limitation, orthopedic/biomechanical evaluation, and assessment of training and running habits.

Junction of the Middle and Proximal Third

FIG 3–2.
A, B (both same patient), Frontal and lateral views demonstrate an intense area of localized augmented uptake in the posterior cortex of the tibia indicating a stress fracture or reaction. *(Continued.)*

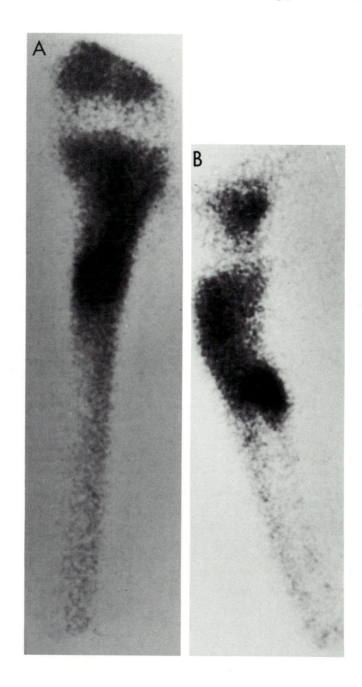

Stress Reaction and/or Fracture—Typical (cont.)

FIG 3–2 (cont.).
C, Localized periosteal new bone formation and endosteal irregularity is evident only on a fluoroscopic spot film obtained tangent to the posterior cortex and not evident on routine films. *(Continued.)*

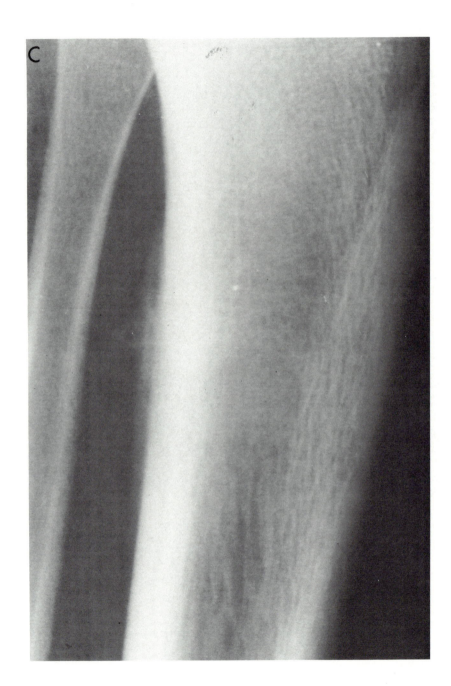

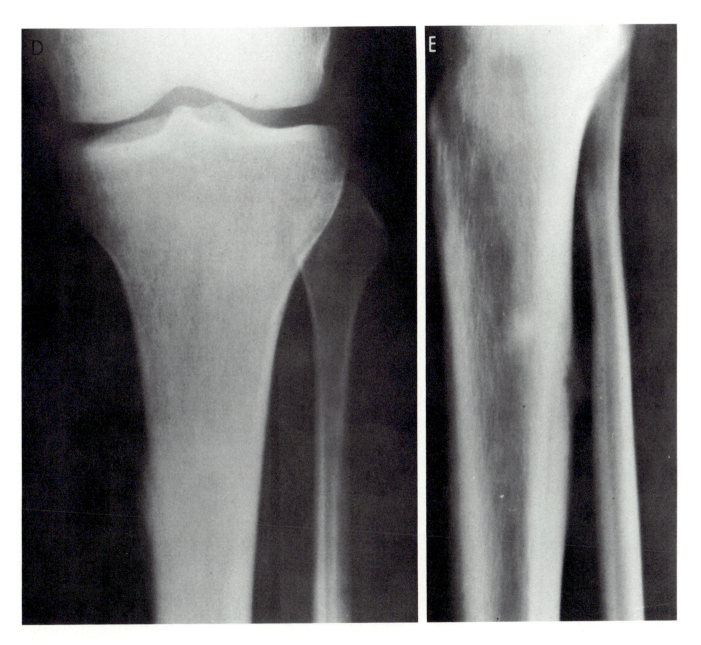

FIG 3–2 (cont.).
D–F (all same patient), Frontal and lateral views
demonstrate localized thickening of the medial
and posterior cortices of the proximal tibia. *(Continued.)*

Stress Reaction and/or Fracture—Typical (cont.)

FIG 3–2 (cont.).
F, On a subsequent lateral view, there is maturity of the localized posterior cortical thickening representing a healed stress reaction. A definitive radiolucent fracture line was never evident. (*Continued.*)

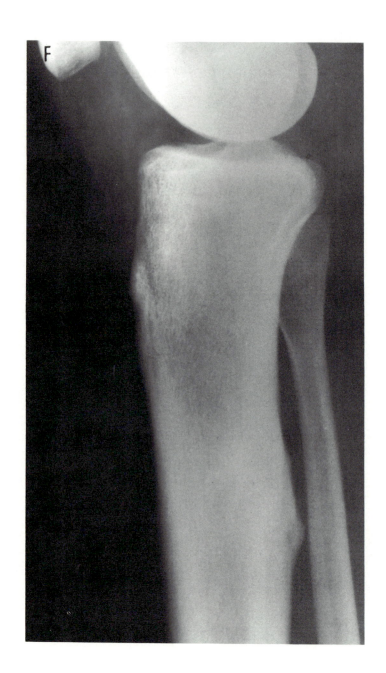

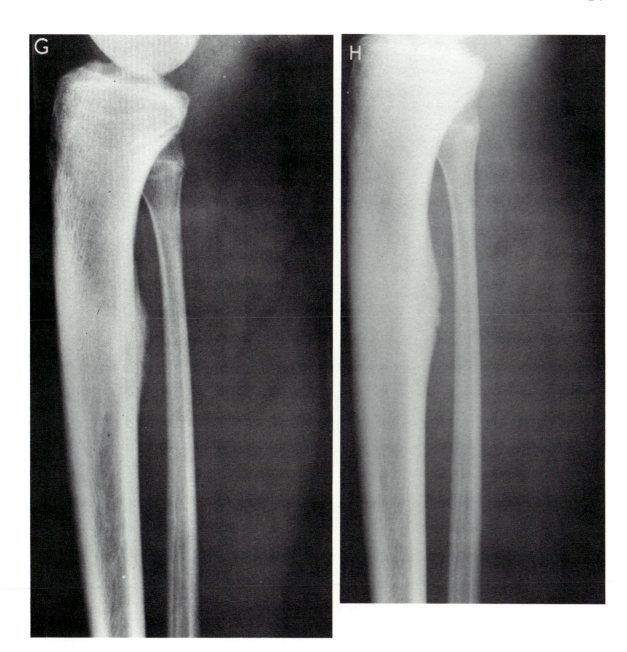

FIG 3–2 (cont.).
G, H (both same patient), There is periosteal and endosteal thickening of the posterior tibial cortex with a serrated irregular periosteal pattern.

H, Subsequent radiograph demonstrates continued endosteal and periosteal reaction; however, the appearance is less aggressive and more typical of a healing stress fracture. A definitive radiolucent fracture line was not evident. *(Continued.)*

Stress Reaction and/or Fracture—Typical (cont.)

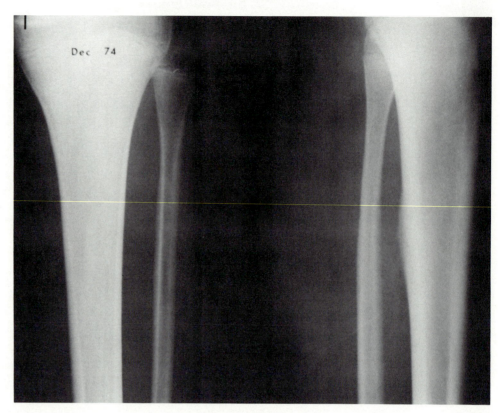

FIG 3–2 (cont.).
I–K (all same patient), 12/74, Localized area of cortical thickening involving both the periosteal and endosteal surfaces is seen on the lateral view. AP view is unremarkable.

J, One month later (1/75) lateral view demonstrates increase in the localized hyperostosis and cortical thickening and the periosteal reaction is evident on the AP view.

K, Two months later (3/75) there is mature periosteal new bone formation. A definitive stress fracture was not identified. However, the bones showed continued response as the patient continued to run despite roentgen findings and pain. (*Continued.*)

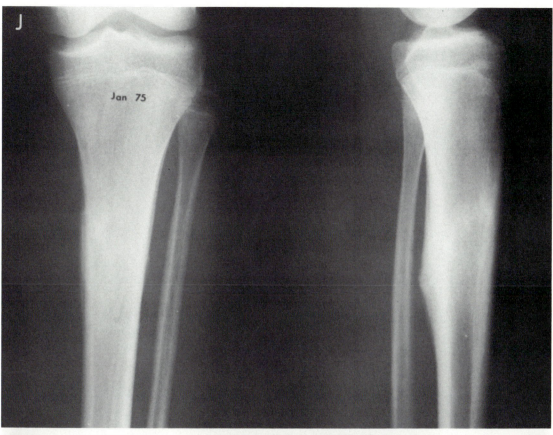

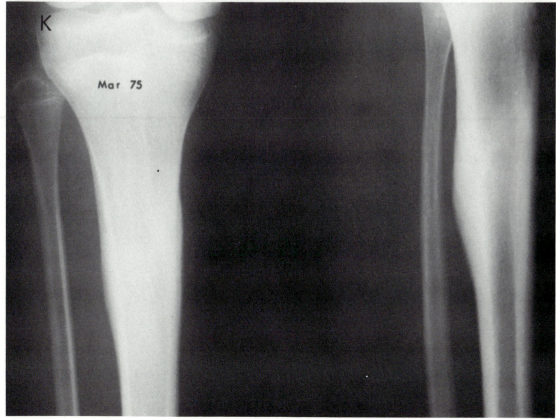

Stress Reaction and/or Fracture—Typical (cont.)

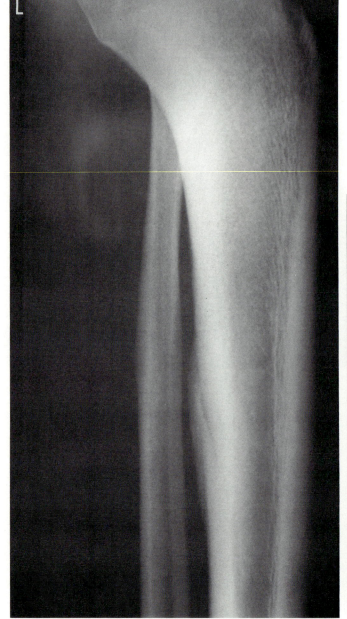

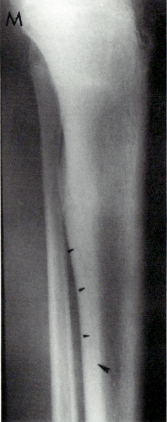

FIG 3–2 (cont.).
L, An oblique radiolucent fracture line is present within the area of posterior cortical thickening at the junction of the proximal and middle third of the tibia. There is irregularity of both the endosteal and periosteal surfaces.
M, A radiolucent stress fracture has propagated distally within an area of cortical thickening *(arrowheads)*. *(Continued.)*

FIG 3–2 (cont.).
N,O (both same patient), A radiolucent fracture line is identified within the localized area of hyperostosis of the posterior medial cortex. The horizontal radiodensity identified crossing the marrow cavity represents endosteal new bone formation, osteoblastic activity, and collapsed fractured trabeculae.

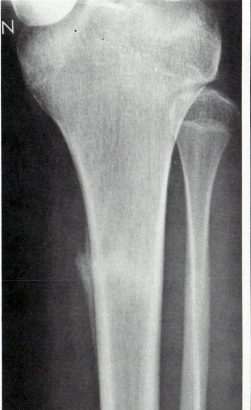
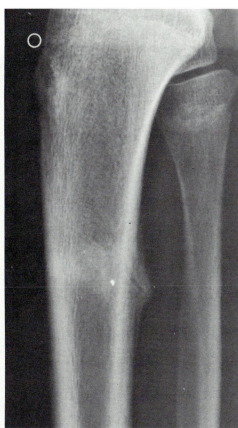

P, Q (both same patient), On the routine lateral view, there is localized cortical thickening and a broad zone of radiodensity crossing the marrow cavity of the proximal tibia.
Q, On an overpenetrated tomogram, a radiolucent fracture line is seen extending into the marrow cavity. The broad zone of sclerosis obscures the fracture on the routine views but on the tomogram the sclerosis is seen to border the fracture margin and indicates a delayed or nonunion. (Continued.)

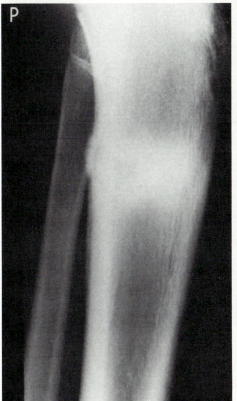
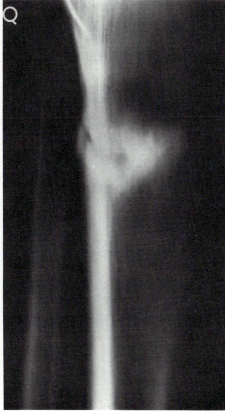

Stress Reaction and/or Fracture—Typical (cont.)

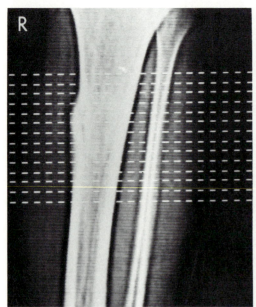

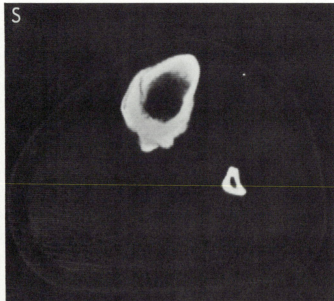

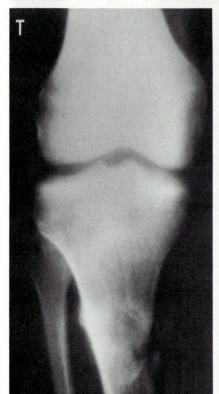

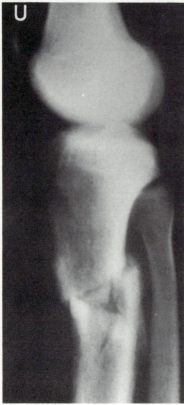

FIG 3–2 (cont.).
R, S (both same patient), Scout film for a computed tomogram (CT) demonstrates localized periosteal and endosteal reaction of the medial cortex of the proximal tibia.
S, Axial image demonstrates a radiolucent fracture line within the localized area of cortical hyperostosis. The fracture involves only the medial cortex and does not extend into the marrow cavity.

T,U (both same patient), and **V,W** (both same patient) (facing page), Frontal and lateral views of two patients demonstrate stress fractures that propagated completely across the tibial shaft. (Permission for **C,L,M,P,Q** granted courtesy of Pavlov H, Torg JS, Hersh A, et al: The roentgen examination of runners' injuries. *RadioGraphics* 1981; 1:17–34.)

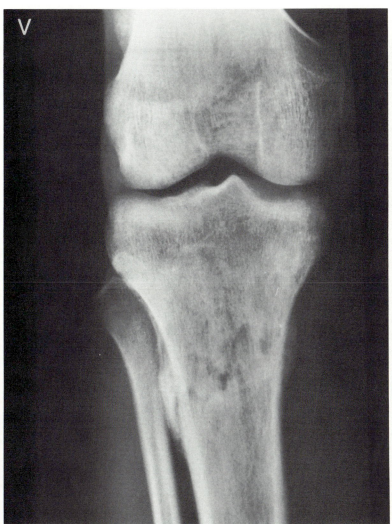

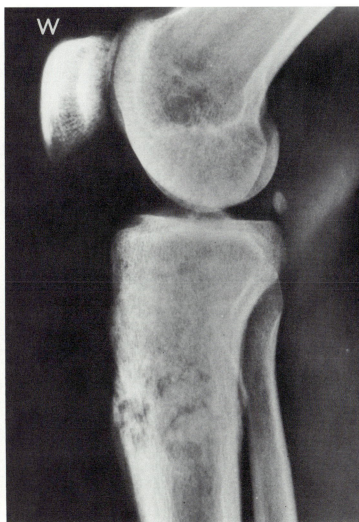

Stress Reaction and/or Fracture—Typical

Junction of the Middle and Proximal Third

REMEDY   Activity limitation, orthopedic/biomechanical evaluation, and assessment of training and running habits. *Complete fracture:* cast immobilization.

Stress Reaction and/or Fracture—Atypical

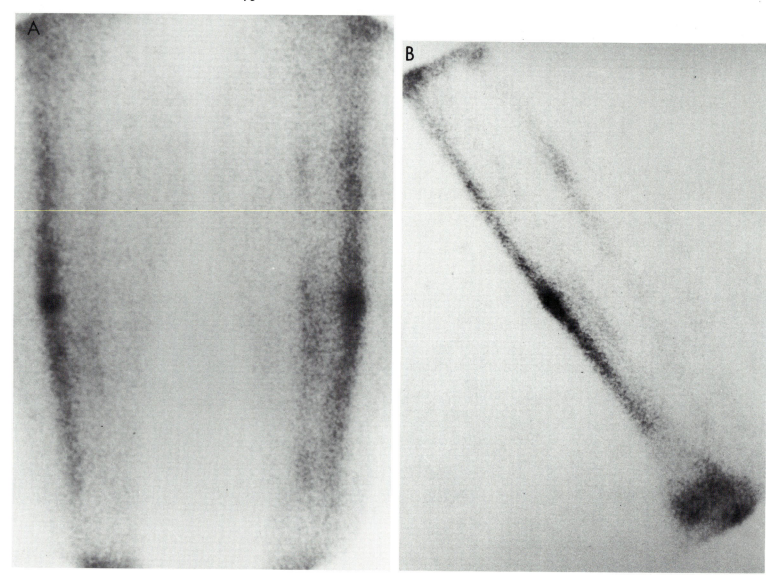

Anterior Cortex—Solitary Lesion

FIG 3–3.
A, B (both same patient), Symmetric areas of augmented isotope uptake in the midshaft of both tibias.
B, the lateral scan view, the uptake is confined to the anterior cortex. (Permission for **A,B** granted courtesy of Pavlov H, Torg JS, Hersh A, et al: The roentgen examination of runners' injuries. *RadioGraphics* 1981; 1:17–34.) *(Continued.)*

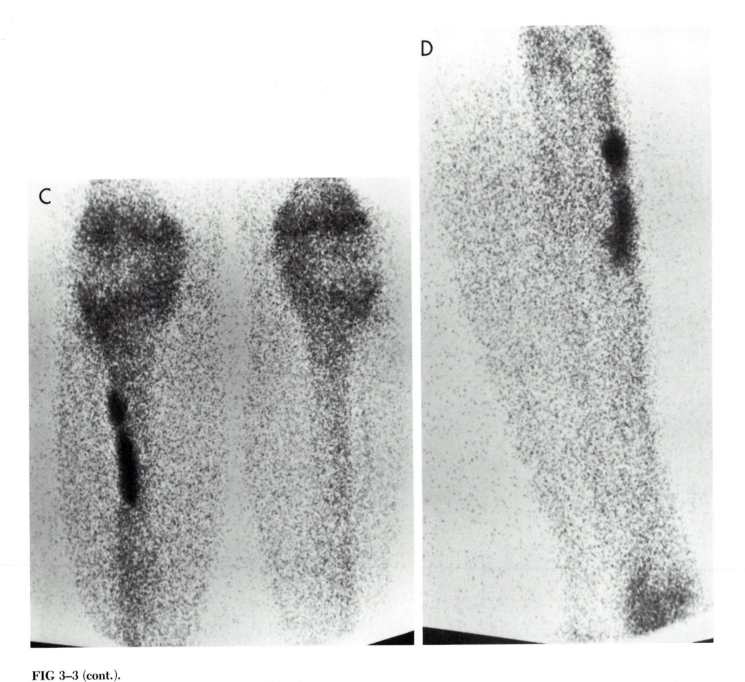

FIG 3–3 (cont.).
C,D (both same patient), Elongated area of localized augmented isotope uptake involving the lateral aspect of the anterior cortex of the right tibia at the junction of the proximal and middle thirds. *(Continued.)*

Stress Reaction and/or Fracture—Atypical (cont.)

FIG 3–3 (cont.).
E,F (both same patient), Frontal and lateral view demonstrate a localized area of hyperostosis in the lateral anterior aspect of the tibia *(arrow)*. A small horizontal radiolucent fracture line is seen on the lateral view *(open arrow)*.

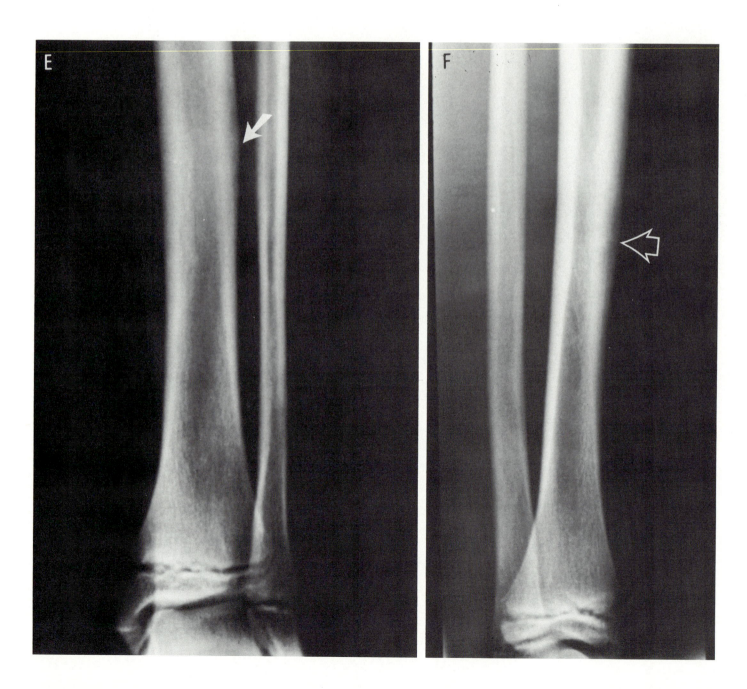

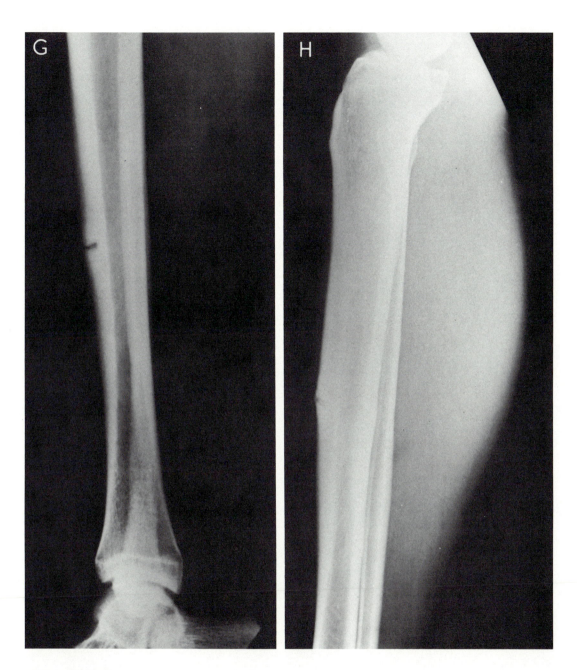

FIG 3–3 (cont.).
G,H,I (**I** appears on following page), Three examples of nonunion, the "dreaded black line:" a
horizontal radiolucent fracture confined to the
cortical hyperostosic area of the anterior tibial
cortex. The fracture is completely surrounded by
sclerotic bone and represents a nonunion. *(Continued.)*

Stress Reaction and/or Fracture—Atypical (cont.)

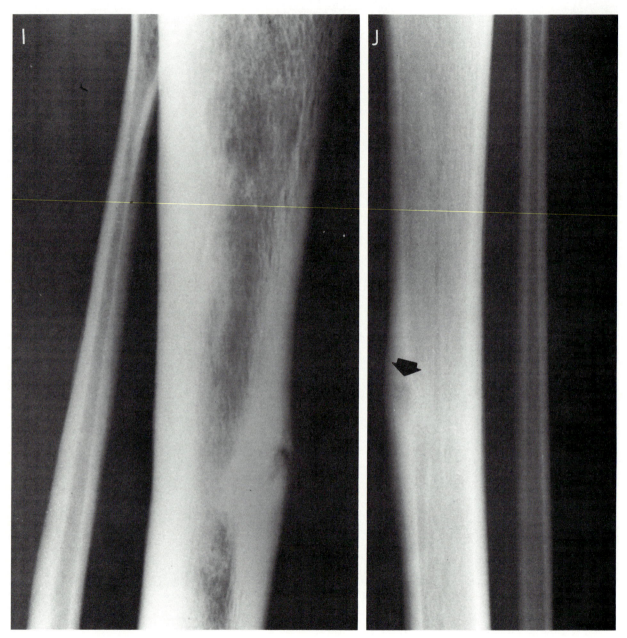

FIG 3–3 (cont.).
J, There is a vague ovoid radiolucency *(arrow)* within the localized hyperostosic area of the anterior cortex. *(Continued.)*

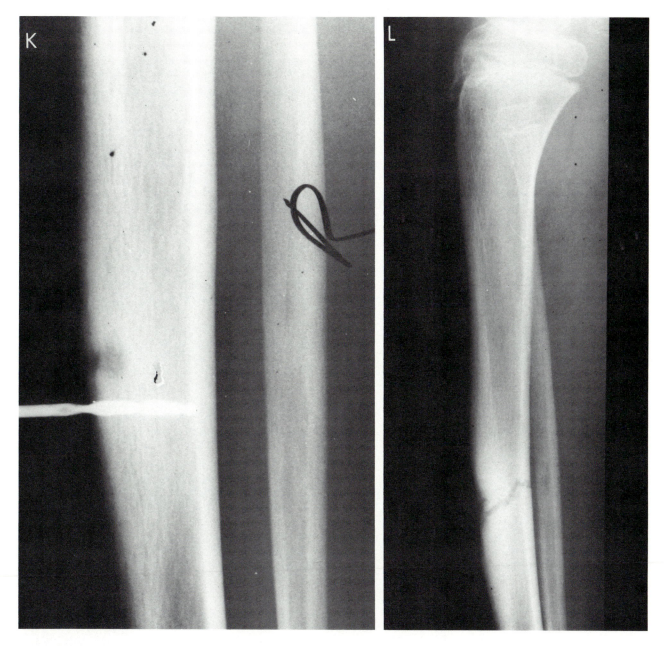

FIG 3–3 (cont.).

A biopsy (**K**) was performed to rule out an osteoid osteoma, infection (Brodies abscess), or an intracortical osteogenic sarcoma. Following the biopsy, (**L**) the tibia fractured completely. This case demonstrates the importance of establishing the diagnosis on the basis of the history and x-ray findings. In addition to problems of a fracture through the stress riser created by the biopsy, interpretation of the fracture callus specimen can be misinterpreted as a malignant process.

Stress Reaction and/or Fracture—Atypical

Anterior Cortex—Solitary Lesion

REMEDY Activity limitation, orthopedic/biomechanical evaluation, and assessment of training and running habits.

Stress Reaction and/or Fracture—Atypical (cont.)

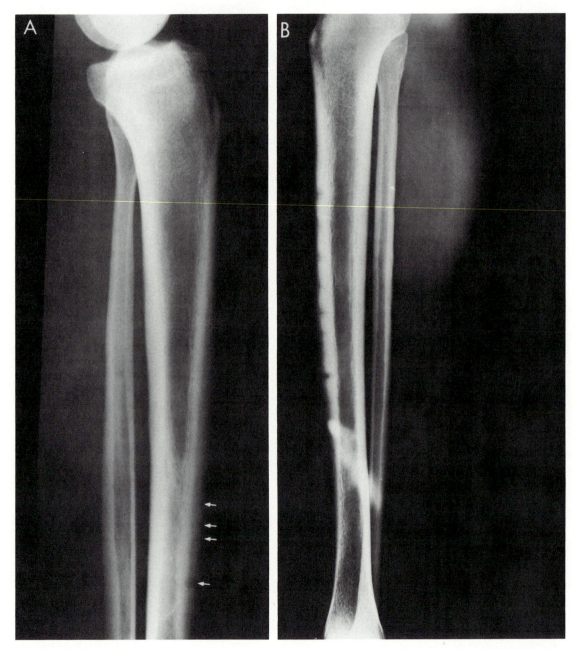

Anterior Cortex—Multiple Lesions

FIG 3–4.
A,B, There are multiple horizontal radiolucent lines *(arrows)* within a thickened anterior cortex. These lines represent stress fractures at various stages of healing. (Permission for **A** granted courtesy Pavlov H, Torg JS, Hersh A, et al: The roentgen examination of runners' injuries. *RadioGraphics* 1981; 1:17–34.) *(Continued.)*

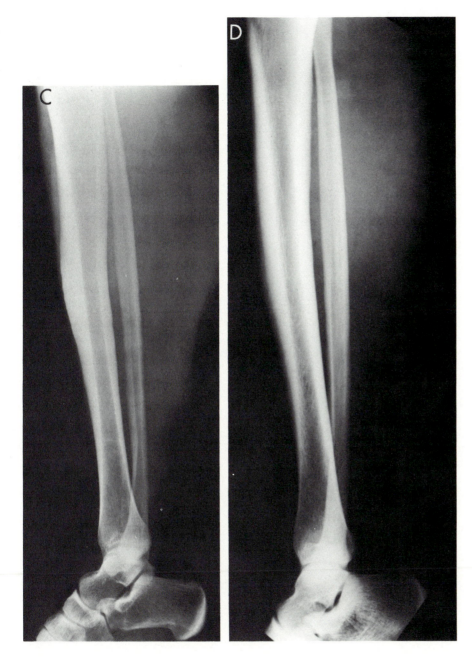

FIG 3–4 (cont.).
C,D, Two examples of stress reactions or healed stress fractures demonstrated by the elongated area of cortical hyperostosis involving the anterior cortex of the midtibia. The posterior cortex is normal.

Stress Reaction and/or Fracture—Atypical

Anterior Cortex—Multiple Lesions

REMEDY: Activity limitation, orthopedic/biomechanical evaluation, and assessment of training and running habits.

Shin Splints

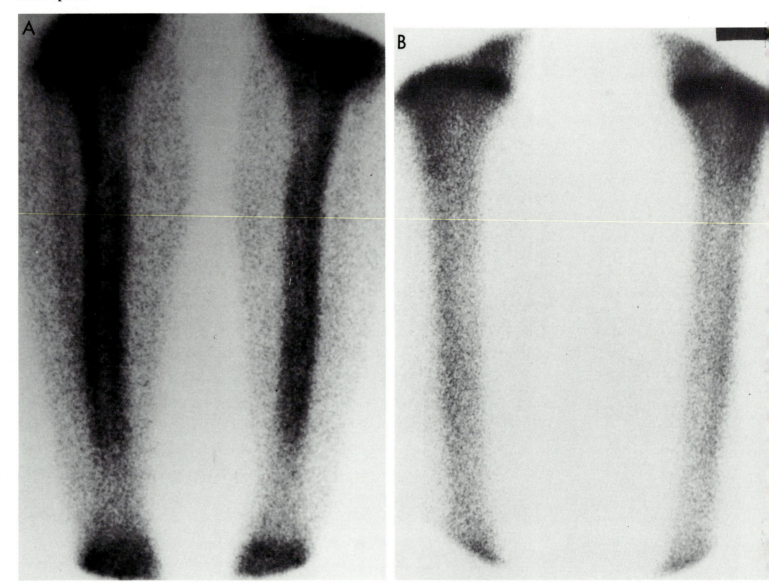

FIG 3–5.
A, Frontal radionuclide bone scan demonstrates augmented isotope uptake involving the middle two thirds of the tibias bilaterally, consistent with shin splints. **B,** Frontal view demonstrates the normal radionuclide bone scan pattern with progressive decreasing uptake from the proximal to distal tibia. *(Continued.)*

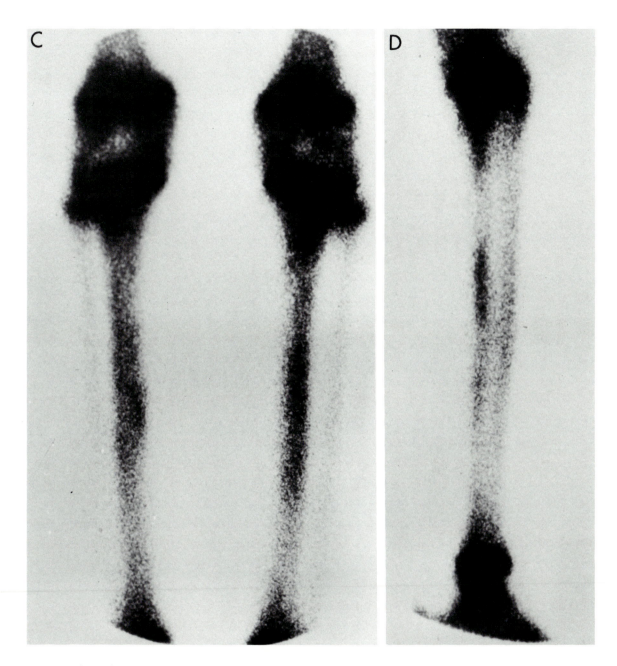

FIG 3–5 (cont.).
C,D (both same patient), Localized uptake in the
posterior and medial cortex with "normal" radiographs is consistent with shin splints. It is important for the *medial* aspect of the tibia to be
placed against the gamma camera. (Ref: Holder
LE, Michael RH: The specific scintigraphic pattern of "shin splints" in the lower leg. *J Nucl
Med* 1984; 25:865.) *(Continued.)*

Shin Splints (cont.)

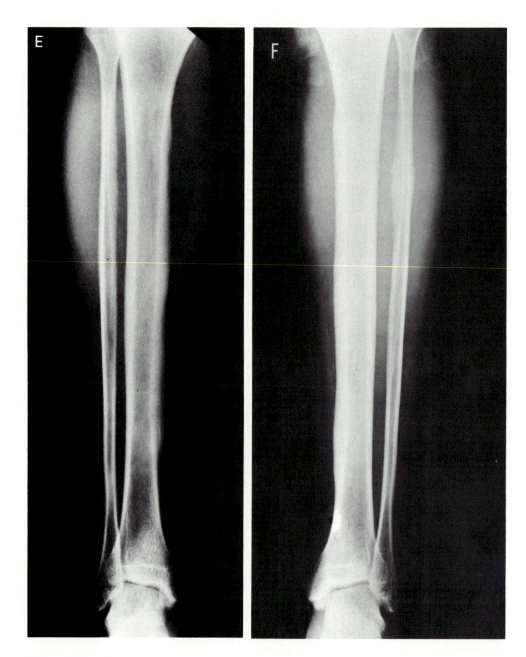

FIG 3–5 (cont.).
E–G (all same patient), Multiple areas of localized cortical thickening results in a wavy contour
of the tibia and proximal fibula secondary to multiple stress reactions and fractures at various
stages of healing.

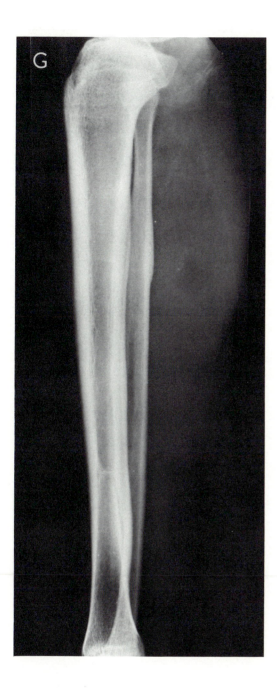

Shin Splints

REMEDY   Activity limitation, orthopedic/biomechanical evaluation and assessment of training and running habits.

FIBULA

Salter I Fracture

FIG 3–6.
A,B (both same patient), Initial examination demonstrates soft tissue swelling adjacent to the lateral malleolus; the fibular epiphyses has a normal appearance. Soft-tissue swelling adjacent to an open epiphysis is always suggestive of a Salter I fracture.

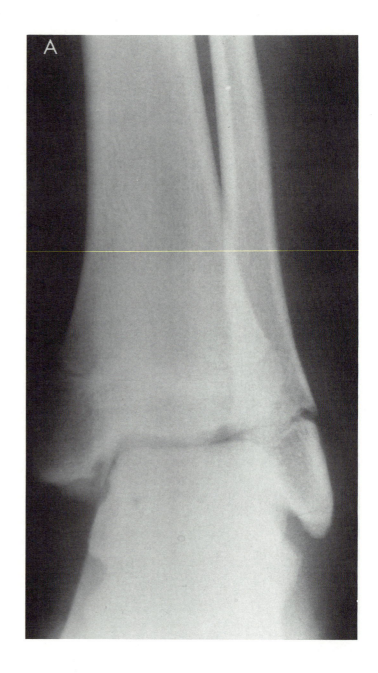

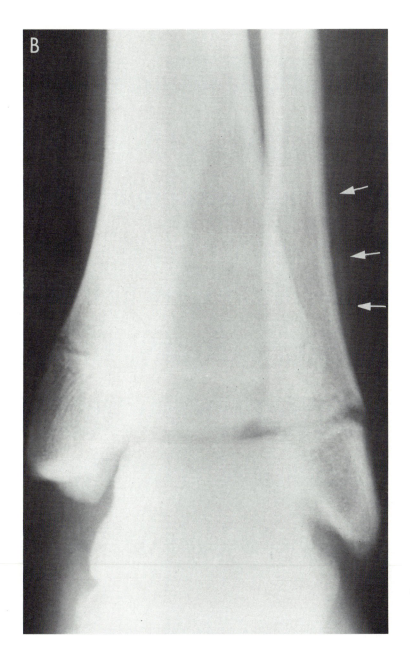

B, Repeat examination 10 days later demonstrates periosteal new bone formation *(arrows)* adjacent to the lateral fibular cortex, confirming the presence of a Salter I fracture. (Permission for **A,B** granted courtesy of Pavlov H, Torg JS, Hersh A, et al: The roentgen examination of runners' injuries. *RadioGraphics* 1981; 1:17–34.)

Salter I Fracture

REMEDY   Non-weight-bearing cast.

Stress Reaction and/or Fracture—Fibula

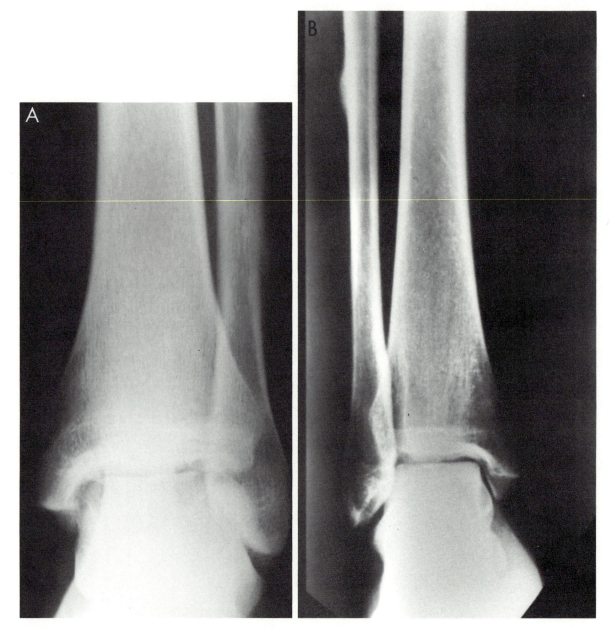

FIG 3–7.
A,B, Periosteal new bone formation adjacent to the lateral cortex of the fibula without a radiolucent fracture line indicates a stress reaction or healed stress fracture. *(Continued.)*

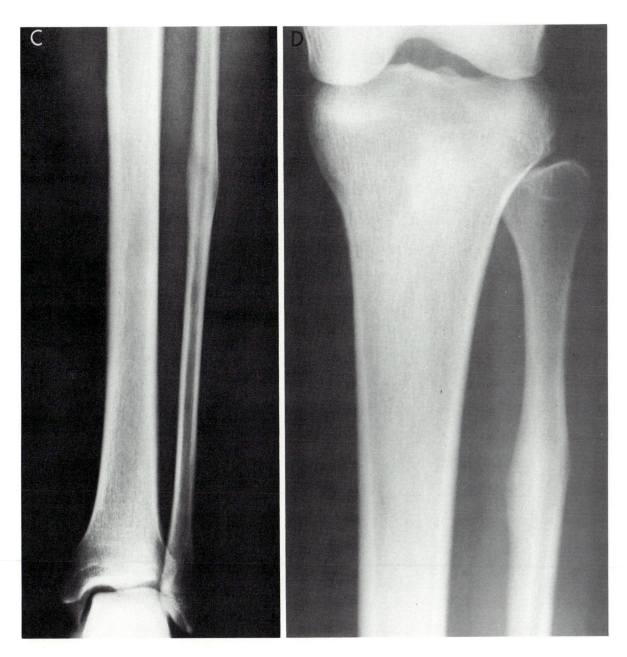

FIG 3–7 (cont.).
C,D, Two examples of fibular stress reactions.
There is localized periosteal and endosteal thickening at various sites on the fibular shaft. The
fracture line is not seen. *(Continued.)*

Stress Reaction and/or Fracture—Fibula

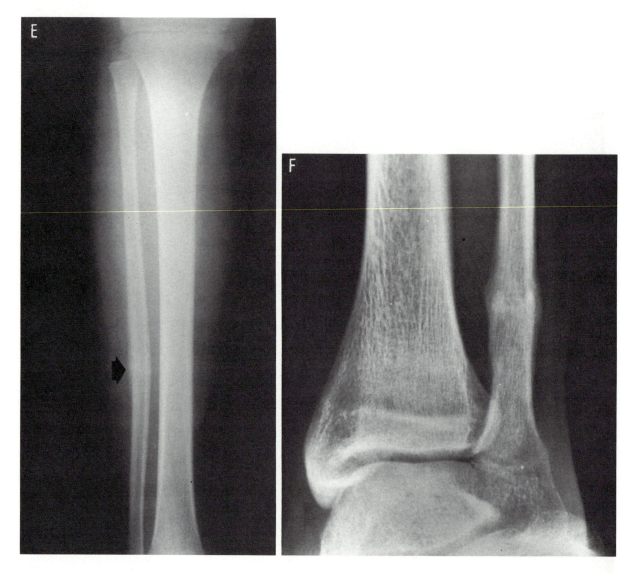

FIG 3–7 (cont.).
E,F, Two examples of healing stress fractures
that completely crosses the fibula. *(Continued.)*

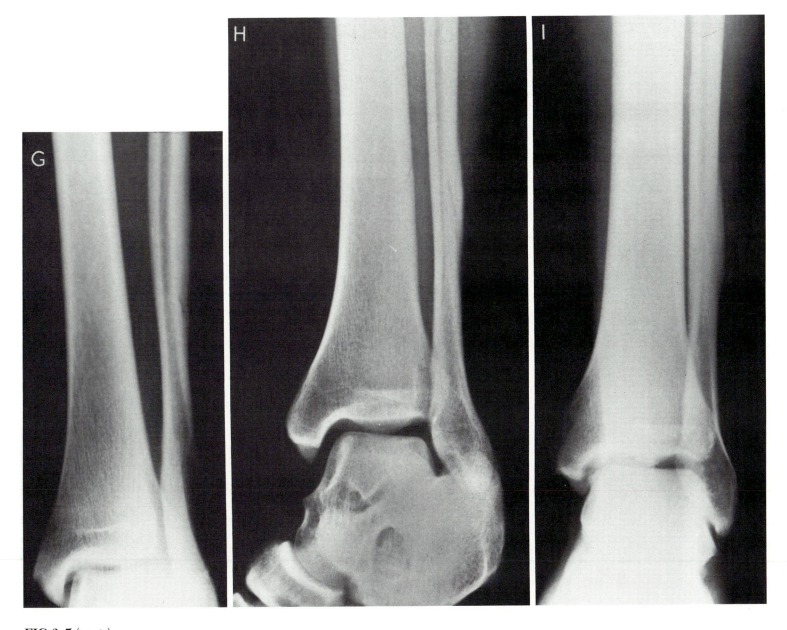

FIG 3–7 (cont.).
G,H, I (all same patient), Progression of a healing stress fracture. **G,** Initially, there is a radiolucent stress fracture within the localized area of lateral cortical thickening. **H,** The fracture line has propagated proximally but there is loss of definition of the radiolucent fracture line indicating healing. **I,** There is complete healing with a resultant thick lateral fibular cortex.

Stress Reaction and/or Fracture—Fibula

REMEDY   Activity limitation, orthopedic/biomechanical evaluation, and assessment of training and running habits.

CHAPTER 4

The Knee

TIBIOFEMORAL JOINT

Degenerative Osteoarthritis

FIG 4–1.
Early changes are demonstrated by narrowing of
the medial joint compartment with proliferative
osteophytes along the medial and lateral joint
margins and on the tibial spines.

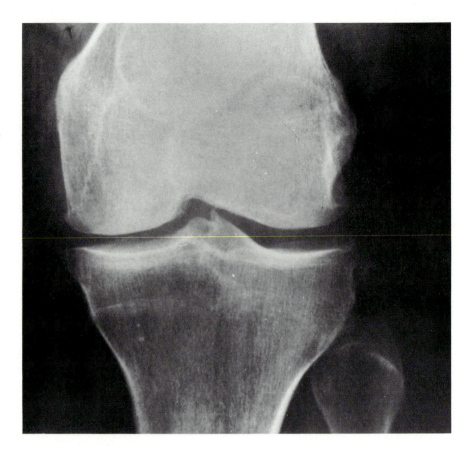

Degenerative Osteoarthritis

REMEDY If symptomatic and/or effusion, arthroscopic examination and la-
vage are indicated. Rule out intra-articular lesions, i.e., degenerative meniscal tears. If there is associated pain, activity limitation is indicated.

TIBIA

Stress Reaction and/or Fracture—Tibia

FIG 4–2.
The proximal end of the tibia, like the distal end, is cancellous bone.
A, The horizontal zone of radiodensity beneath the medial tibial plateau at the metaphyseal diaphyseal junction represents a typical stress fracture of cancellous bone. *(Continued.)*

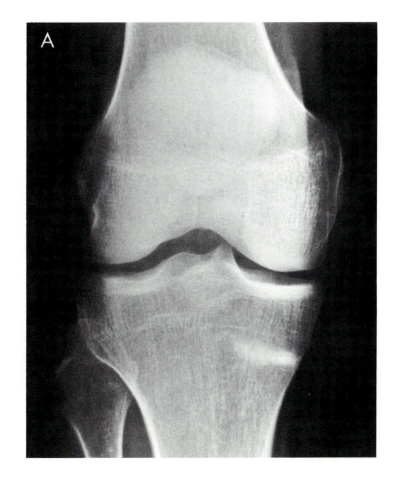

Stress Reaction and/or Fracture—Tibia (cont.)

FIG 4–2 (cont.).
B,C (both same patient), The fuzzy horizontal density beneath the medial tibial plateau on the oblique and lateral views (*arrows*) typifies a stress fracture.

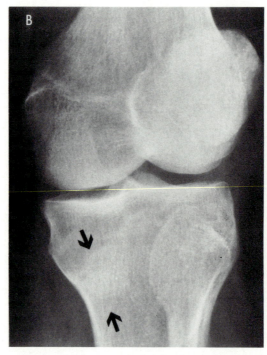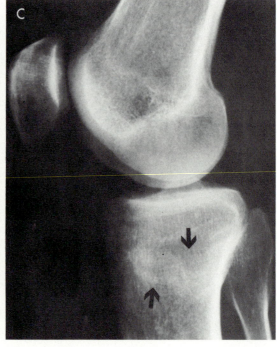

Stress Reaction and/or Fracture—Tibia

REMEDY   Activity limitation, orthopedic/biomechanical evaluation, and assessment of training and running habits.

Osteochondritis Dissecans/Necrosis

FIG 4–3.

A,B (both same patient), Arthrotomogram (anteroposterior [AP] and lateral) demonstrates intact articular cartilage overlying the osseous notch defect in the lateral tibial plateau *(arrows)*. On the lateral view, a well-corticated osseous density *(arrow)* is identified within the lesion. Incidentally, there is a nonossifying fibroma in the posterior aspect of the proximal tibial metaphysis. (Ref: Lotke PA, and Ecker ML: Osteonecrosis-like syndrome of the medial tibial plateau. *Clin Orthop* 1983; 176:148–153.)

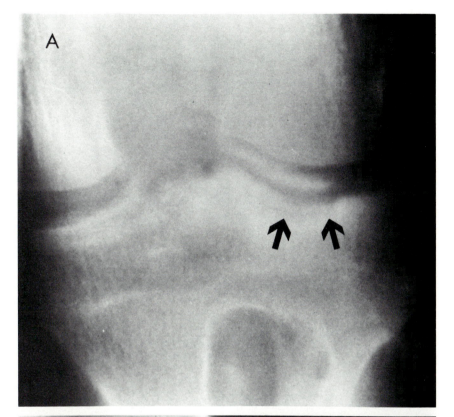

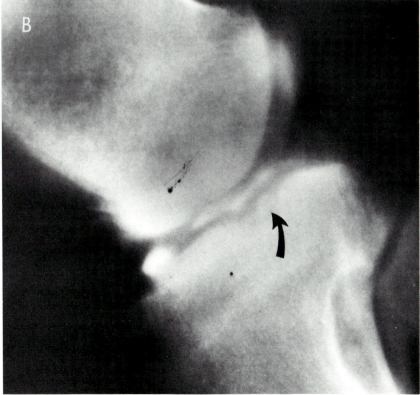

(Remedy appears on the following page.)

Osteochondritis Dissecans/Necrosis

REMEDY   If associated with pain and/or effusion, activity limitation. If symptoms are disabling, non-weight-bearing on crutches is indicated.

Osteochondral Fracture/Avulsion of the Anterior Cruciate Ligament

FIG 4–4.
Arthrotomogram (lateral view) demonstrates an avulsed osteochondral fragment *(arrows)* at the insertion site of the anterior cruciate ligament. The contrast completely surrounds the osteochondral fragment, which indicates it is loose.

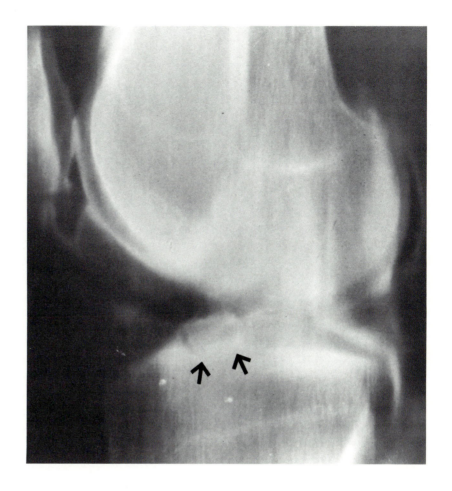

Osteochondral Fracture/Avulsion of the Anterior Cruciate Ligament

REMEDY

In the child: immobilization in a non-weight-bearing cylinder cast with the knee in extension till fracture heals.
In the adult: open reduction and internal fixation.

Tumors

Aneurysmal Bone Cyst

FIG 4–5.
An eccentric lytic aneurysmal bone cyst in the proximal medial tibia with a pathologic nondisplaced fracture through the medial cortex *(arrow)*. Patient developed pain during a marathon at 18 miles and had to stop running.

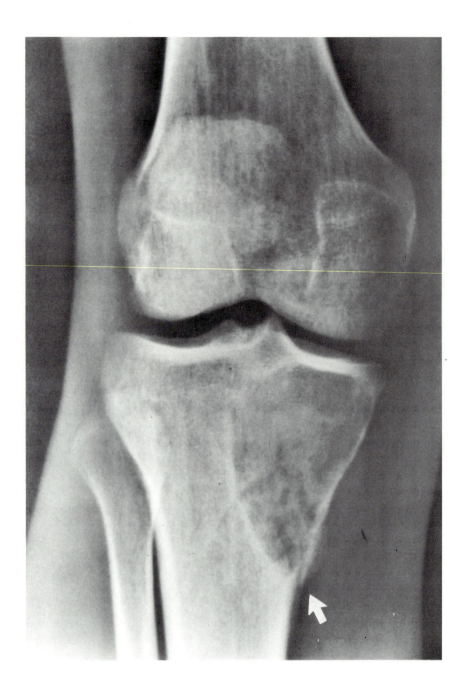

Aneurysmal Bone Cyst

REMEDY   Curettage and autogenous graft.

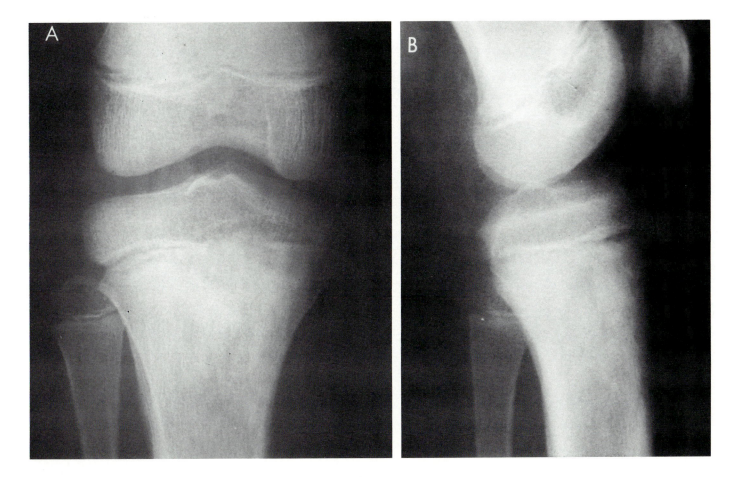

Ewing's Sarcoma

FIG 4–6.
A,B (both same patient), Frontal and lateral
views demonstrate increased density and loss of
the normal bony trabeculae and periosteal reaction in the proximal metaphysis. The lesion stops
at the growth plate, radiographically.

Ewing's Sarcoma

REMEDY   Radiation, chemotherapeutic and/or surgical protocol.

Tumors (cont.)

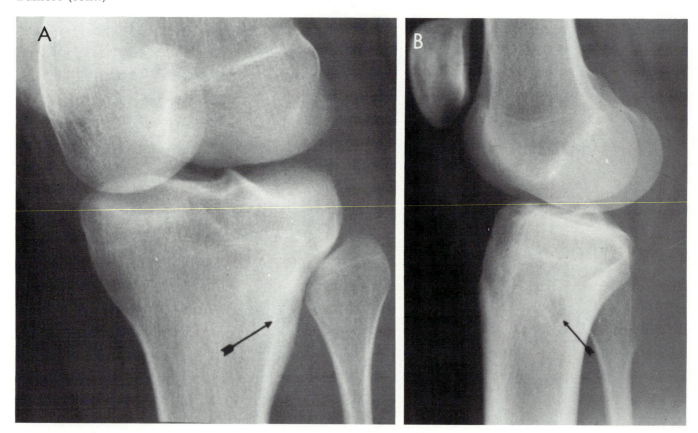

Osteoid Osteoma

FIG 4–7.
A,B (both same patient), Oblique and lateral
views demonstrate an ovoid lucent nidus *(arrow)*
in the lateral cortex. (Permission granted courtesy of Pavlov H, Torg JS, Hersh A, et al: The
roentgen examination of runners' injuries.
RadioGraphics 1981; 1:17–34.)

Osteoid Osteoma

REMEDY   Surgical excision.

PATELLA

Normal Variants

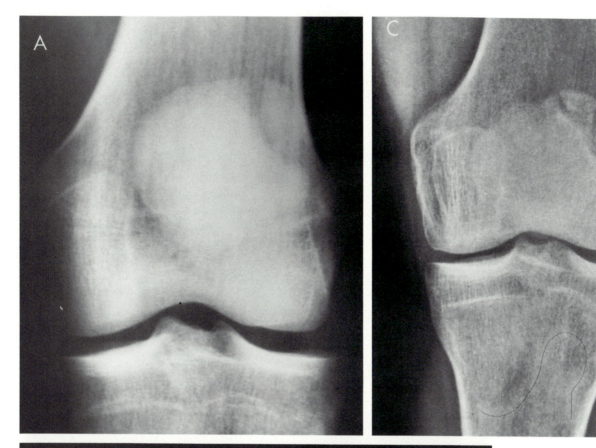

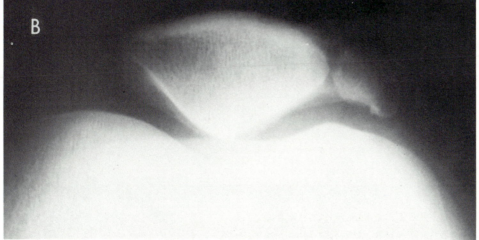

FIG 4–8.
A,B (both same patient), Typical bipartite patella on AP and Merchant views. There is a separate corticated fragment at the supralateral aspect. **C,** Multipartite patella with several well-corticated fragments at the supralateral aspect. *(Continued.)*

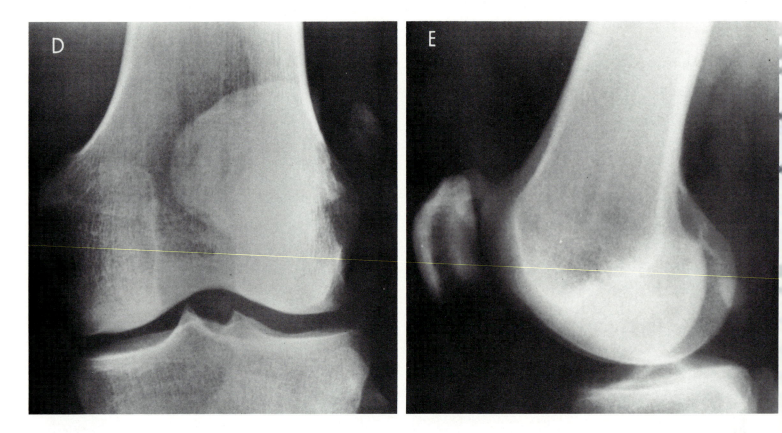

FIG 4–8 (cont.).
D,E (both same patient), Frontal and lateral
view demonstrate a bipartite patella with lateral
displacement of the supralateral fragment.

Normal Variants

REMEDY   If symptomatic, isometric exercise program, ice, and activity
limitation. If unresponsive to conservative measurement, excision of bipartite fragment should be considered.

Chondromalacia Patella

Arthrographic demonstration of the posterior articular cartilaginous surface of the patella.

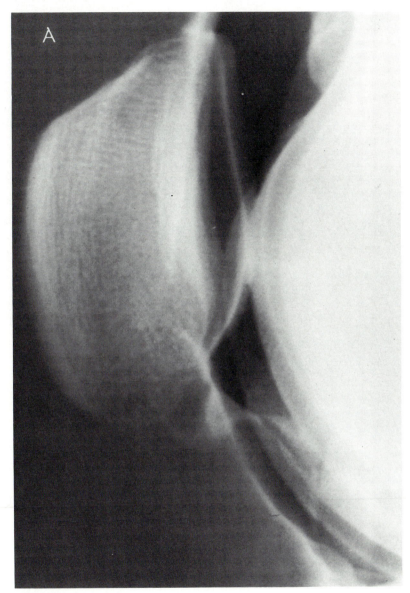

FIG 4–9.
A, Normal. *(Continued.)*

Chondromalacia Patella (cont.)

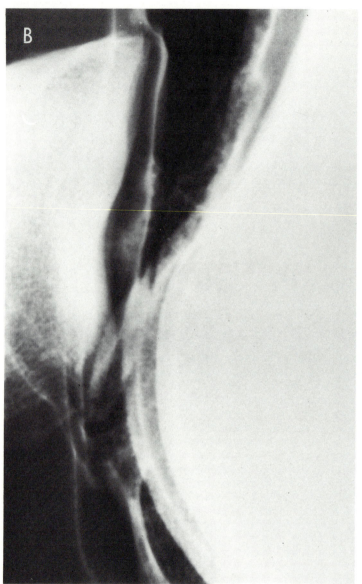

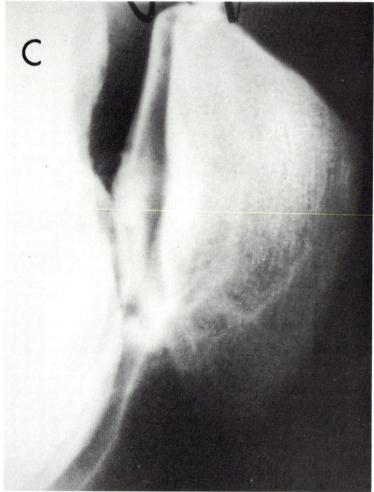

FIG 4–9 (cont.).
B,C, Increased radiodensity in the midportion of
the patellar cartilage that indicates fibrillation
and degeneration changes, classic of early chondromalacia. (Permission for **A,C** granted courtesy
of Pavlov H, Schneider R: Extrameniscal abnormalities as diagnosed by knee arthrography.
Radiologic Clinics of North America. 1981;
19:287.) *(Continued.)*

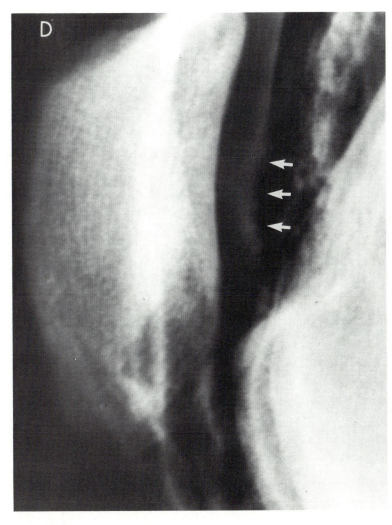

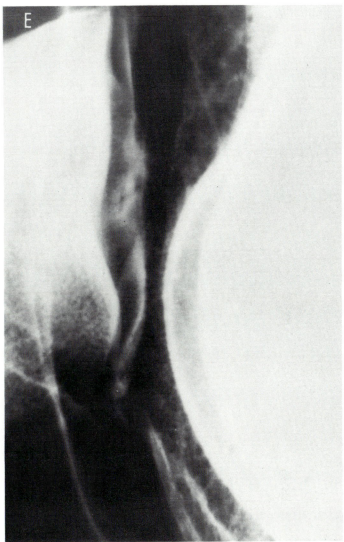

FIG 4–9 (cont.).
D, Ulceration in the midportion of the posterior articular cartilage *(arrows).*

E, Fracture of the cartilage and early cartilage erosion. (Permission for **E** granted courtesy of Pavlov H: Sports related knee injuries, in Taveras JM (ed): *Radiology/Diagnosis/Imaging/Intervention.* Philadelphia, JB Lippincott Co, 1986.) *(Continued.)*

Chondromalacia Patella (cont.)

FIG 4–9 (cont.).
F, Thinning of the articular cartilage over the superior half of the patella *(arrows).*

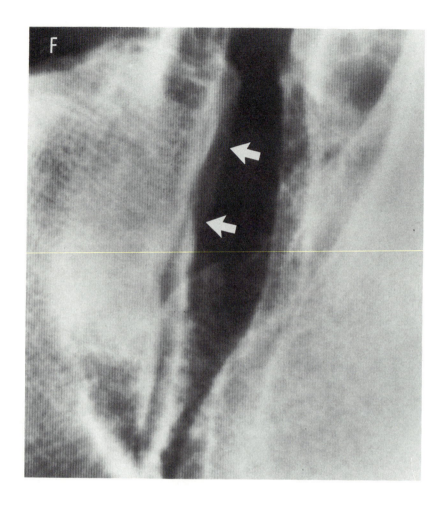

Chondromalacia Patella

REMEDY

Conservative management: ice, isometric quadriceps strengthening exercises, aspirin, patellar support.
Surgical management: (1) arthroscopic shaving of cartilaginous defects; (2) lateral retinacular release in those knees with tight retinacular structures; and (3) extensor realignment and/or Maquet procedure for those knees with recurrent subluxation/dislocation associated with extensor malalignment.

Patellar Tracking

FIG 4–10.
A, Normal patellar femoral alignment is the congruence angle *(oad)* and is normally less than + 16 degrees. (Ref: Merchant AC, Mercer RL, Jacobsen RH, et al: Roentgenographic analysis of patello-femoral congruence. *J Bone Joint Surg* 1974; 56A:1391–1396.)

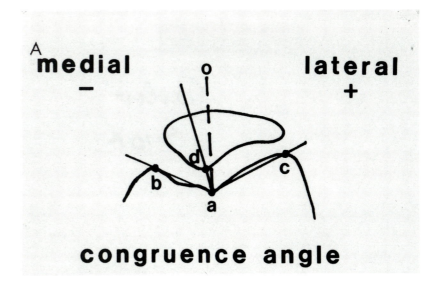

B, The Merchant view, performed with the cassette below the knees and the knees flexed 45 degrees, best demonstrates the congruence angle and detection of abnormal patellar tracking. (Permission for **A,B** granted courtesy of Insall JN: *Surgery of the Knee.* New York, Churchill Livingstone, 1984.) *(Continued.)*

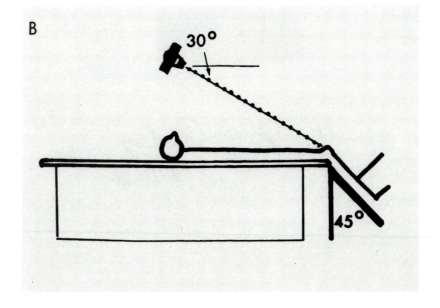

Patellar Tracking (cont.)

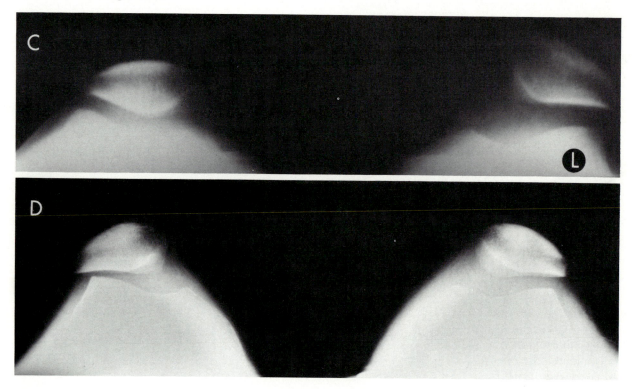

FIG 4–10 (cont.).
C, Merchant view demonstrates subluxation of the left patella. **D,** Bilateral lateral subluxation with narrowing of lateral compartment of the right patellar femoral joint.

Patellar Tracking

REMEDY

Patellar pain and/or chondromalacia that are secondary to patellar femoral tracking abnormalities can be divided into two groups: (1) a conservative exercise regime, and (2) surgery.

Conservtive treatment: in patients with patellar pain syndrome symptoms but without evidence of joint surface pathology, effusion, and/or quadriceps atrophy, management is conservative. Conservative management consists of an isometric quadriceps-strengthening program, instruction about the use of ice after exercise, and a regimen of 600 mg of acetylsalicylic aspirin, 3 to 4 times a day with meals for 6 weeks. The patients are followed clinically by examination for effusion, quadriceps atrophy, and for the presence or absence of the patellar inhibition test. The patellar inhibition test is the inability of the patient to contract the quadriceps with pressure exerted on the superior aspect of the patellar pole distally. In the presence of a positive patellar inhibition, the isometric regimen is followed. After 6 or 12 weeks, when the patellar inhibition test reverts to negative, the patient is placed on a short arc isotonic exercise regimen. In instances where conservative management fails or the patient presents with abnormal patellar tracking associated with effusion and/or quadriceps atrophy, arthroscopic evaluation of the patellar femoral surfaces and the remainder of the joint is indicated.

Surgical treatment: In those patient in whom there is the presence of effusion, quadriceps atrophy, and articular defects associated with tight retinacular structures and no evidence of malalignment, a lateral retinacular release is indicated. In patients with the clinical findings that are associated with hypermobility and passive subluxability/dislocatability of the patella, an extensor realignment procedure is indicated. In children with open epiphysis, a proximal realignment utilizing the vastus medialis advancement is indicated. In patients with closed epiphysis, we prefer a modified Elmslie-Trillat procedure where the tibial tuberosity is also elevated in the manner described by Maquet.

Stress Fracture—Patella

Nondisplaced Stress Fracture

FIG 4–11.
A, (2–80) There is increased density in the anterior surface of patella. However, despite patients symptoms of patellar pain, this is an essentially normal radiograph. **B,** (11–81) A complete nondisplaced fracture through patella at the junction of middle and distal thirds.

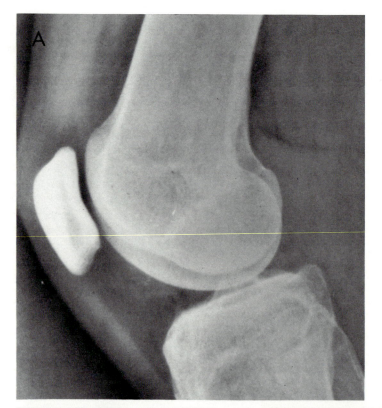

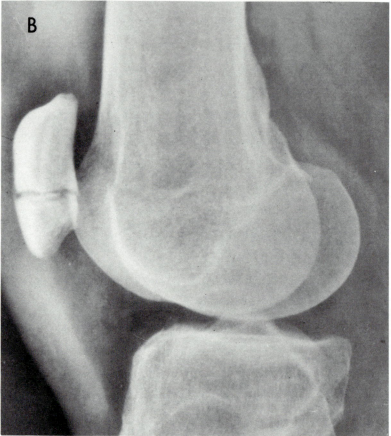

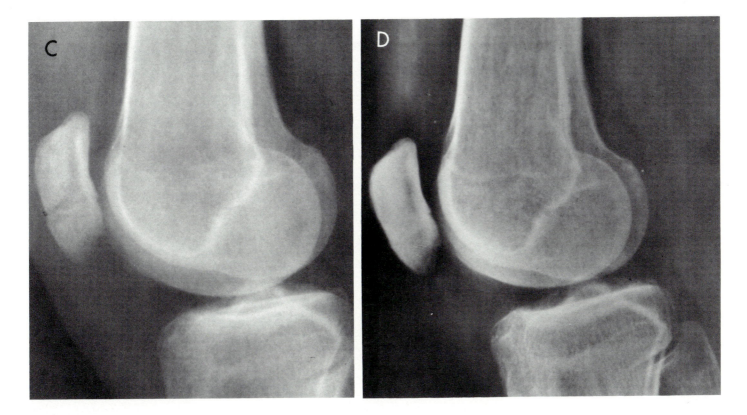

FIG 4-11 (cont.).
C, D, (12–81 and 4–82) Progressive fracture
healing is evident.

Stress Fracture—Patella

REMEDY   Long leg non-weight-bearing cylinder and cast immobilization
                    for 6 weeks.

Stress Fracture—Patella (cont.)

Displaced Stress Fracture

FIG 4–12.
A–C (all same patient; **A** is left knee; **B,C** are right knee), Bilateral complete stress fracture through the patella with distraction of fracture fragments. The quadriceps mechanism is disrupted. (Permission **A–C** granted courtesy of Hensal F, Nelson T, Pavlov H, et al: Bilateral patellar fractures from indirect trauma. A case report. *Clin Orthop* 1983; 178:207.)

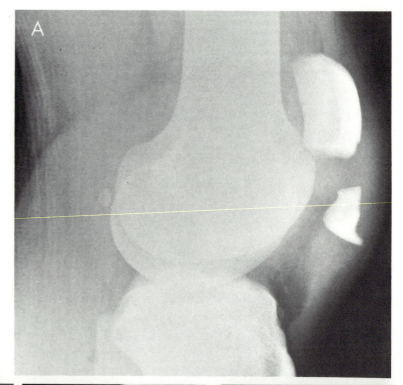

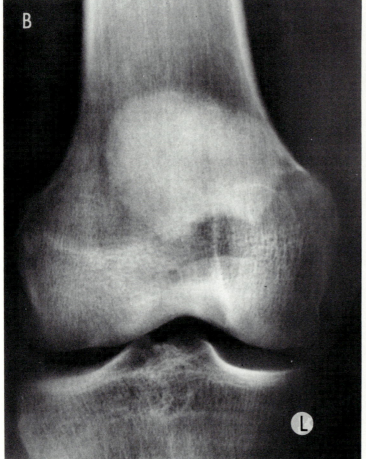

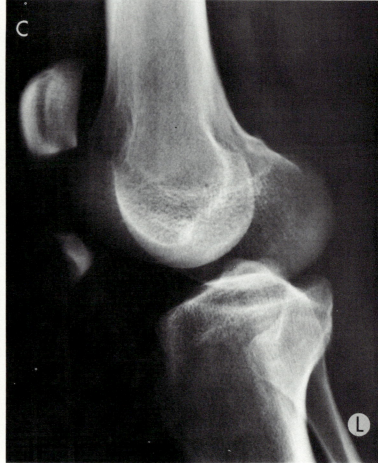

Stress Fracture—Patella

REMEDY   Open reduction, internal fixation, and cast immobilization. **a, b** (both same patient as on prior page, right knee), On AP and lateral views obtained following surgery, tension band wires are demonstrated. (Ref: Lotke PA, Ecker M: Transverse fractures of the patella. *Clin Orthop* 1981; 158:180.)

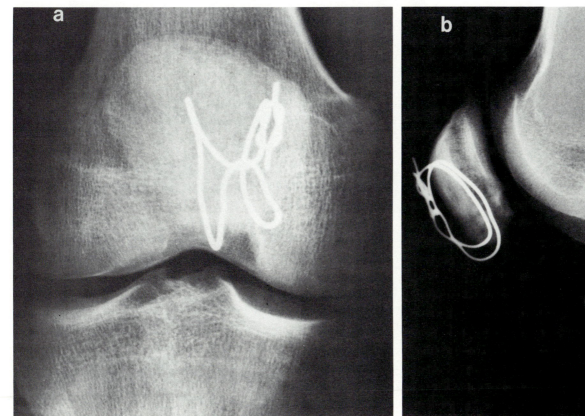
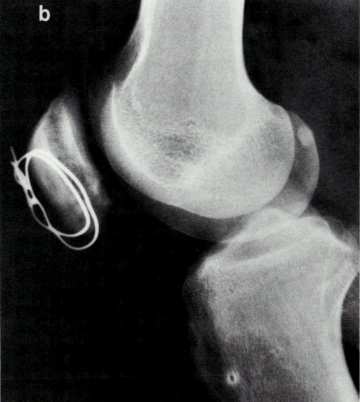

Tumor

Osteoid Osteoma

FIG 4–13.
A, Lateral view demonstrates an oval lucency in the posterior aspect of the patella. **B** (same patient), Radionuclide bone scan of both knees confirms localized isotope uptake in the tumor, best identified on the lateral view *(right)*.

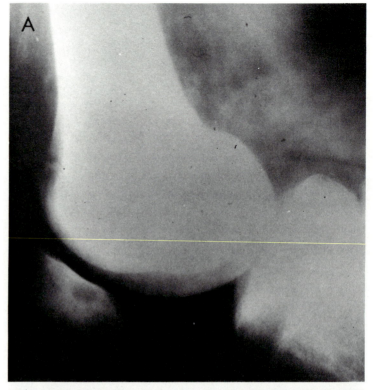

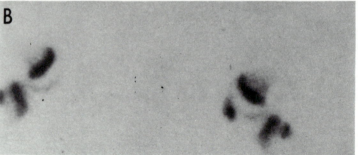

Tumor—Osteoid Osteoma

REMEDY   Surgical excision.

INTRA-ARTICULAR

Joint Effusion

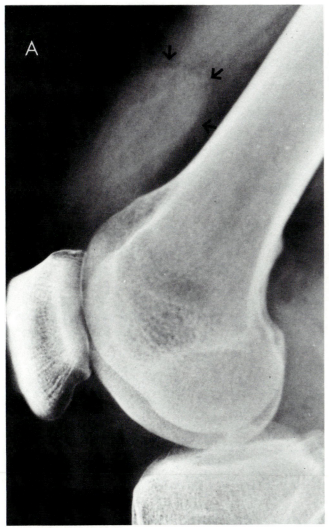

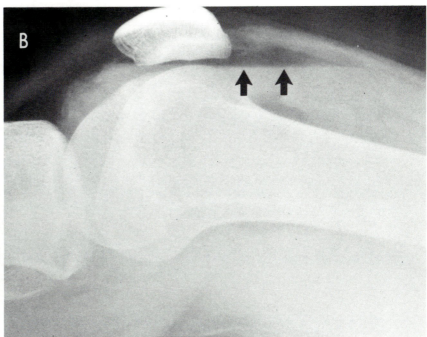

FIG 4–14.
A, Ovoid soft tissue density *(arrows)* posterior to the quadriceps tendon and anterior to the femur indicates blood, pus, or fluid in the joint.
B, A cross-table lateral view demonstrates a fat/fluid level *(arrows)* and indicates there is intra-articular marrow blood secondary to an intra-articular fracture. (Permission for **B** granted courtesy of Torg JS, Pavlov H, Morris VB: Salter-Harris type III fracture of the medial femoral condyle occurring in the adolescent athlete. *J Bone Joint Surg* 1981; 63A:586.)

Joint Effusion

REMEDY Determine etiology of effusion, which may require a diagnostic evaluation that includes clinical, roentgenographic, arthrographic, and/or arthroscopic examination and/or fluid analysis.

Anterior Cruciate Ligament

Normal

FIG 4–15.
A, B, Two examples of an intact anterior cruciate ligament demonstrated by double contrast arthrogram. The contrast/lucent interface of the anterior surface of the anterior cruciate ligament *(arrows)* is "ruler" straight. The anterior cruciate ligament inserts just anterior to the tibial spines and not to the extreme anterior aspect of the tibial plateau. The arthrographic criteria for diagnosing an intact ligament is the same regardless if performed on a horizontal cross-table lateral view (**A**) or a fluoroscopic spot film (**B**). (Ref: Pavlov H: Cruciate ligaments, in Freiberger RF, Kaye JJ (eds): New York, Appleton-Century Crofts, 1979.) *(Continued.)*

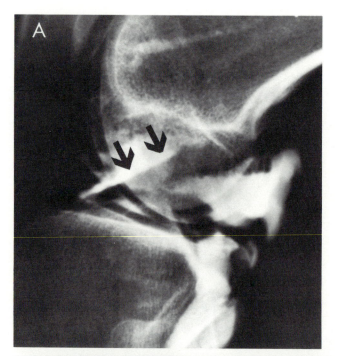

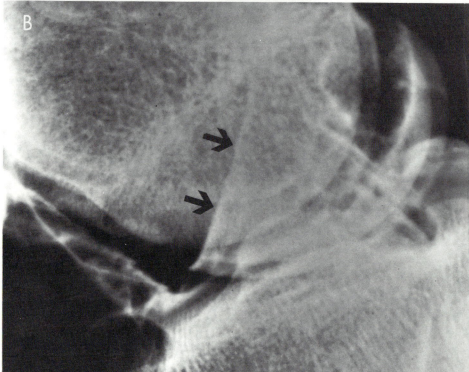

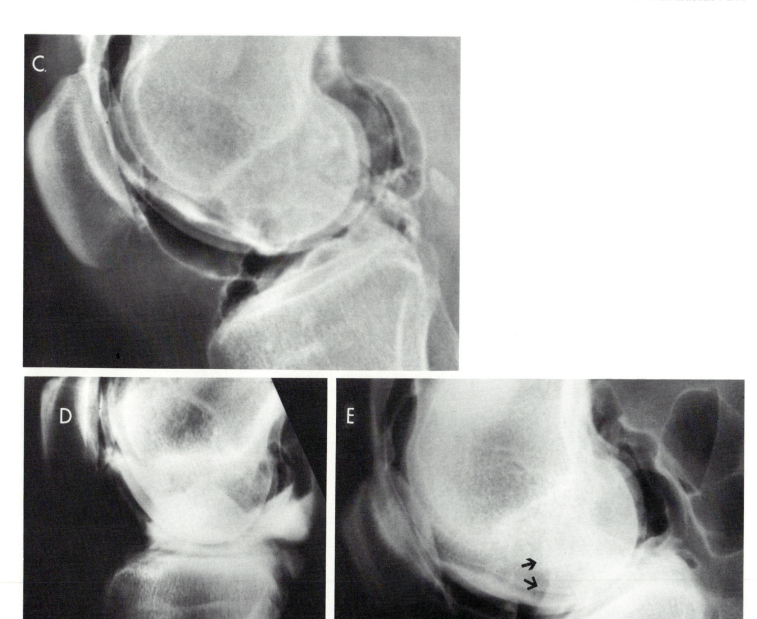

Torn

FIG 4–15 (cont.).
C–E, A torn anterior cruciate ligament on double contrast arthrogram is indicated by either the absence of the ligament
(**C**), pooling of contrast in the region of the anterior cruciate
ligament (**D**), or the acute angulation of an anterior structure
(arrows) (**E**). (Permission for **C–E** granted courtesy Pavlov H,
Warren RF, Sherman MF, et al: The accuracy of double-con-
trast arthrographic evaluation of the anterior cruciate ligament.
A retrospective review of one hundred sixty three knees with
surgical confirmation. *J Bone Joint Surg* 1983; 65A:175–183.)

Anterior Cruciate Ligament

REMEDY:

The Lachman's test is performed to evaluate the anterior cruciate ligament.
a, Lachman's test for anterior cruciate ligament instability is performed with the patient lying supine on the examining table with the involved extremity to the side of the examiner. With the involved extremity in slight external rotation and the knee held between full extension and 15 degrees flexion, the femur is stabilized with one hand and firm pressure is applied to the posterior aspect of the proximal tibia, lifting it forward in an attempt to translate it anteriorly.
b, Position of the examiner's hands is important in performing the test properly. One hand should firmly stabilize the femur, while the other grips the proximal tibia in such a manner that the thumb lies on the anteromedial joint margin.
c, When an anteriorly directed lifting force is applied by the palm and fingers, anterior translation of the tibia in relationship to the femur can be palpated by the thumb. Anterior translation of the tibia associated with a soft or a mushy end point indicates a positive test.

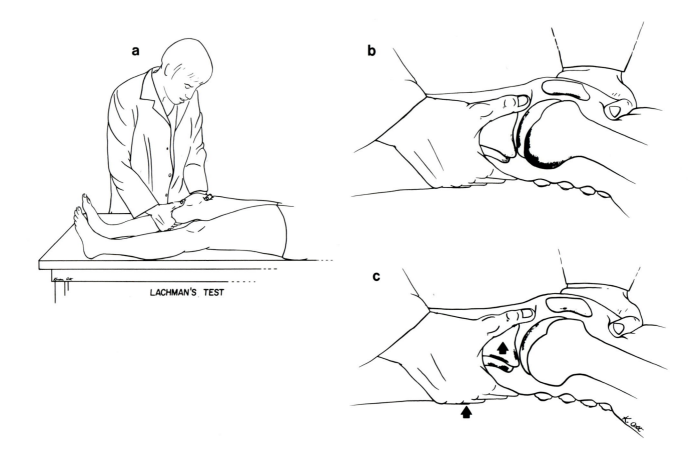

LACHMAN'S TEST

Management of anterior cruciate ligament tears remains controversial. First and foremost, treatment must be individualized to meet the need and demands that the patient will place on the knee. Also, the presence of associated intra-articular and ligamentous injuries must be established and their presence incorporated into the decision-making process.

Isolated tears of the anterior cruciate ligament: in most instances they can be effectively managed with exercises and bracing.

Anterior cruciate ligament disruption associated with derangement of one or both menisci: surgical arthroscopic partial meniscectomy may be effective in giving the patient a more functional knee. In instances where the meniscal lesions are amenable to suture, a concomitant anterior cruciate repair/reconstruction is indicated.

Instability due to associated cruciate and other ligament deficiencies: in the active individual, repair/reconstruction of the torn cruciate is indicated. Although we prefer a modification of the Jones' procedure/reconstruction of the anterior cruciate ligament, the variety and complexity of other surgical alternatives are numerous and beyond the scope of this discussion.

Anterior Cruciate Ligament Avulsion

FIG 4–16.
A–C, Three examples of avulsion of the anterior cruciate ligament insertion: an osseous fragment superior to the tibia, just anterior to the tibial spines *(arrow)*, represents an avulsion injury of the anterior cruciate ligament at its point of insertion. *(Continued.)*

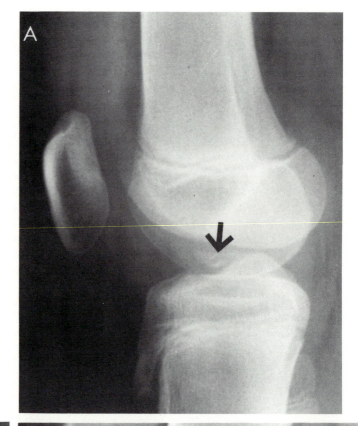

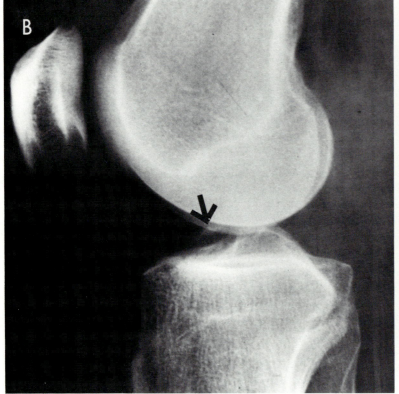

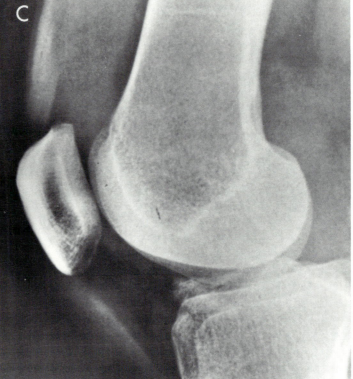

FIG 4–16 (cont.).
D, A fleck of bone in the superolateral aspect of the intercondylar notch *(arrow)* indicates an avulsion of the origin of the anterior cruciate ligament.

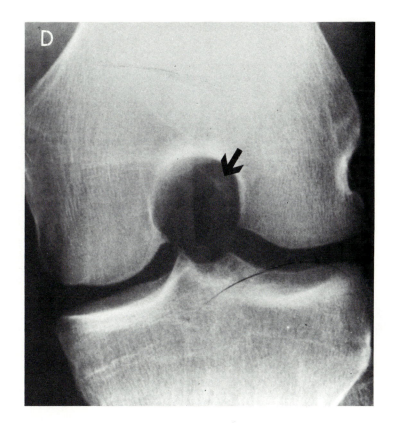

Anterior Cruciate Ligament Avulsion

REMEDY

In the child: immobilization in a non-weight-bearing cylinder cast with the knee in extension till fracture heals.
In the adult: open reduction and internal fixation.

Posterior Cruciate Ligament Avulsion

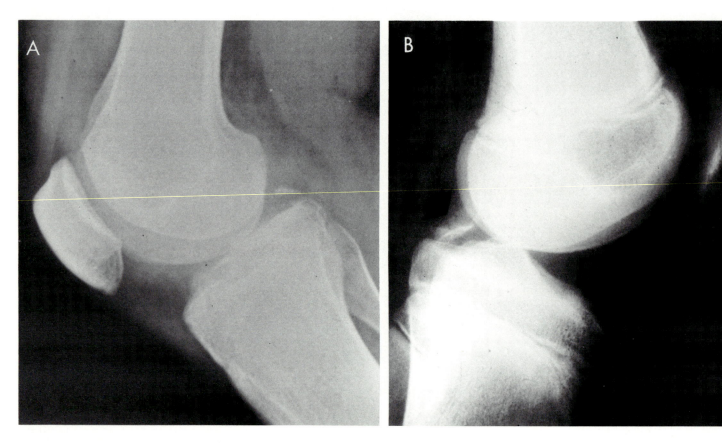

FIG 4–17.
A, B, Two examples: classic appearance of an
avulsion of the posterior cruciate ligament insertion is that of a fleck of corticated bone posteriorly located just proximal to the tibial plateau.

Posterior Cruciate Ligament Avulsion

REMEDY   Surgical repair.

Loose Bodies

FIG 4–18.
A, B (both same patient), Osteochondral loose bodies *(white arrow)* are noted in the posterolateral joint compartment and most probably originated from the sclerotic osteochondral defect *(black arrow)* in the medial femoral condyle. *(Continued.)*

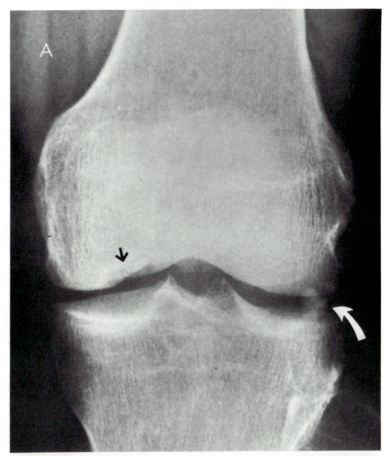

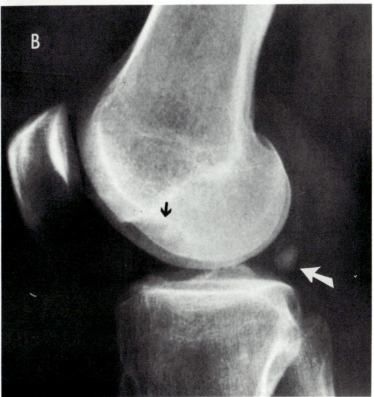

Loose Bodies (cont.)

FIG 4–18 (cont.).
C, D (both same patient), Osteochondral loose bodies in the posteromedial joint compartment. *(Continued.)*

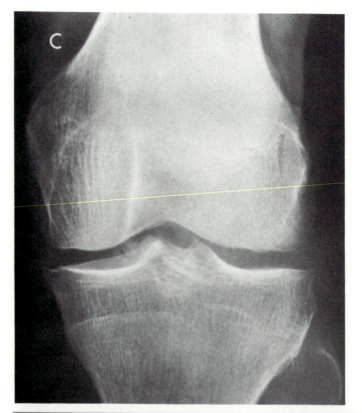

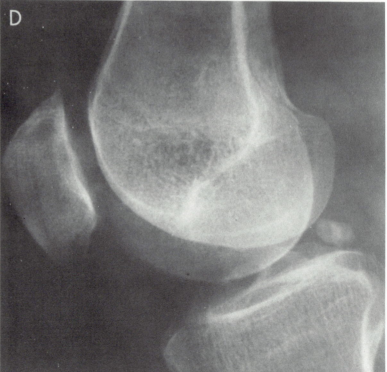

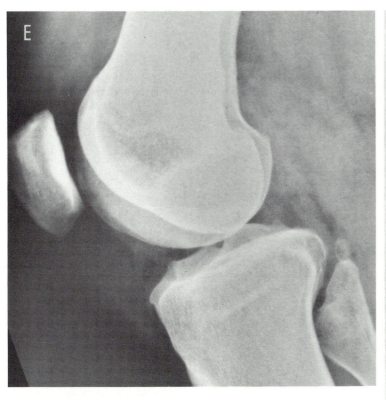

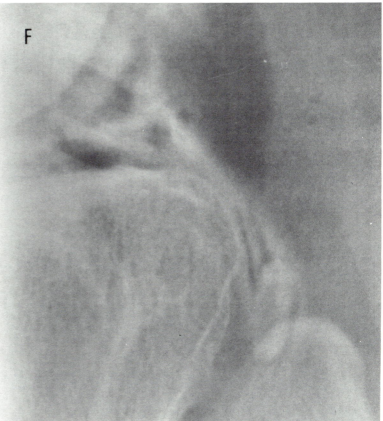

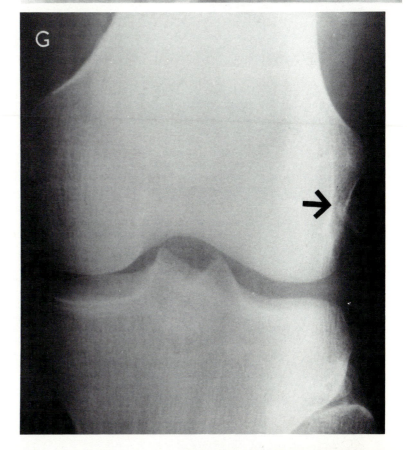

FIG 4–18 (cont.).
E, A well-corticated osseous body posterior to the tibia near the fibular head. **F** (same patient as **E**), On arthrography, the body is identified within the popliteal bursa. This should not be confused with a fabella or cyamella. A fabella is a sesmoid in a lateral head of the gastrocnemius muscle and seen to project over the lateral femoral condyle on the AP view and posterior to the condyles on the lateral view. A cyamella *(arrow)* is a sesamoid in the popliteus tendon and located with the notch on the lateral aspect of the femoral condyle (**G**). *(Continued.)*

Loose Bodies (cont.)

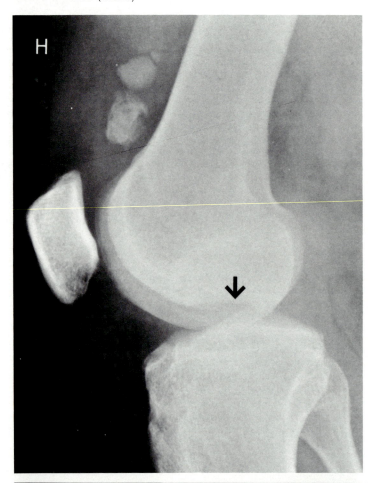

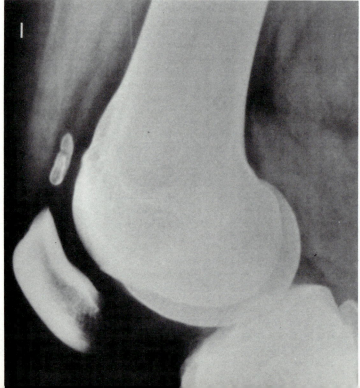

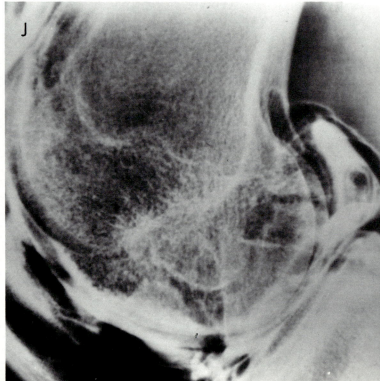

FIG 4–18 (cont.).
H, Two large osteochondral bodies are present in the suprapatellar bursa, originating from the osseous defect in the femoral condyle *(arrow)*. **I,J** (both same patient), Lateral view demonstrates a large osteochondral body in the supracondylar bursa. **J,** On the arthrogram, the osteochondral body is surrounded by contrast and located in the posterior joint compartment. The arthrogram confirms the loose body is intra-articular and freely moves in the joint *(Continued.)*

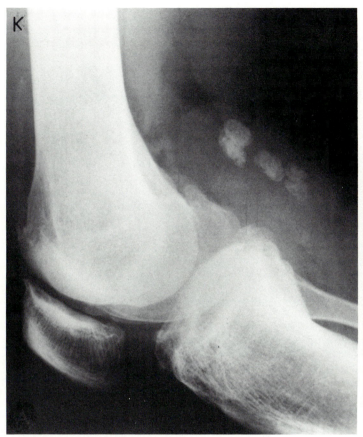

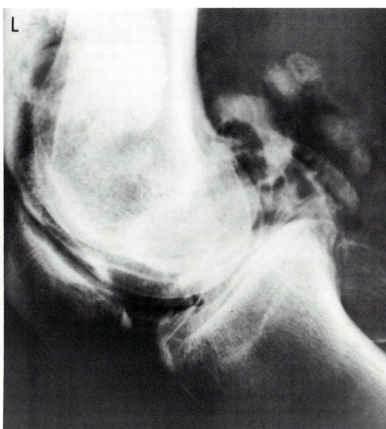

FIG 4–18 (cont.)
K, L (both same patient), multiple osteochondral loose bodies are present posterior to the joint.
L, Arthrography confirms that these bodies are intra-articular and within a popliteal cyst. (Permission for **K, L** granted courtesy of Pavlov H, Schneider R: Extrameniscal abnormalities as diagnosed by knee arthrography. *Radiol Clin North Am* 1981; 19:287.)

Loose Bodies

REMEDY   Intra-articular loose bodies can generally be removed utilizing arthroscopic surgical techniques. Osteochondral bodies in the popliteal bursa that are symptomatic require an open procedure for removal.

Meniscal Ossicle

FIG 4–19.

Loose bodies must be distinguished from a meniscal ossicle, an osseous body embedded within a post-meniscectomy meniscal fragment. The meniscus can be identified by arthrography that will document the location of the osseous body within the meniscal substance. In this instance, the ossicle is in the posterior horn remnant of the medial meniscus.

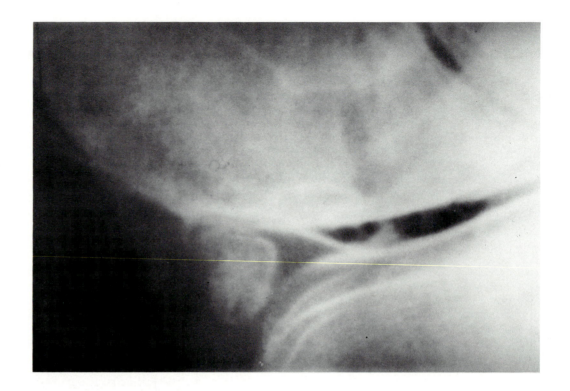

Meniscal Ossicle

REMEDY Surgical arthroscopic removal of meniscal remnant.

Hoffa's Disease—Fat Pad Necrosis

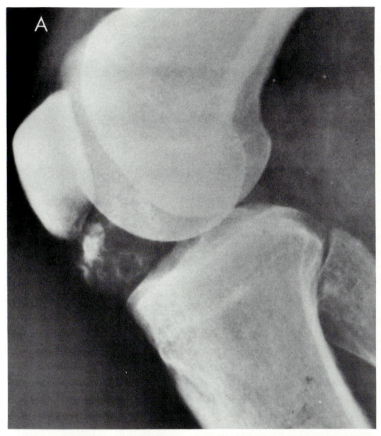

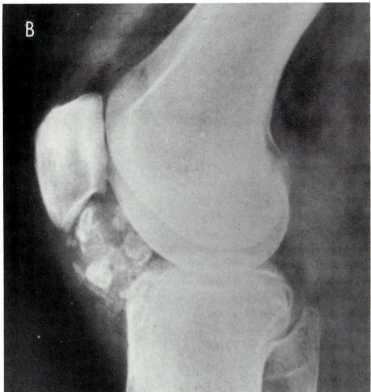

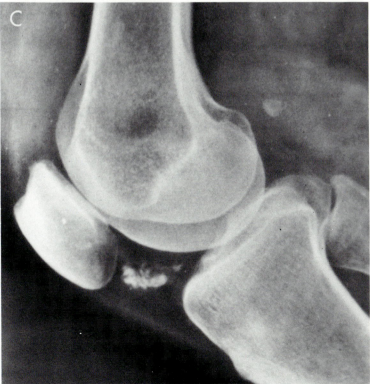

FIG 4–20.
A–C, Three examples: Calcific densities within the fat pad indicates necrosis of the fat pad. These densities must be differentiated from intra-articular loose bodies. (Permission for **C** granted courtesy of Pavlov H: Sports related knee injuries; in Taveras JM (ed): *Radiology/Diagnosis/Imaging/Intervention.* Philadelphia, JB Lippincott Co, 1986.) (Ref: Hoffa A: The influence of the adipose tissue with regard to the pathology of the knee joint. JAMA 1904; 43:795; and Smillie I.S.: Diseases of the Knee, ed. 2. New York, Churchill Livingstone, 1980, p 161.)

(Remedy appears on the following page.)

Hoffa's Disease—Fat Pad Necrosis

REMEDY   If symptomatic, surgical excision.

Popliteal Cyst—Baker's Cyst

Normal

FIG 4–21.
A, B (both same patient), The normal posterior joint compartment is demonstrated on arthrography when the knee is flexed (**A**). This compartment is not seen when the knee is extended (**B**). *(Continued.)*

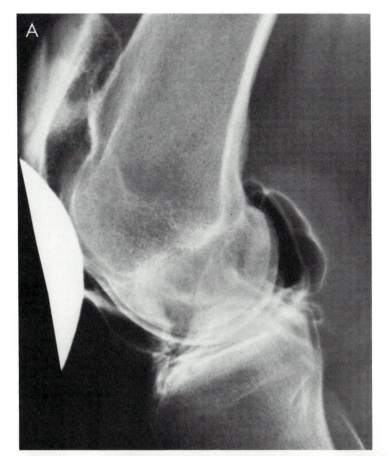

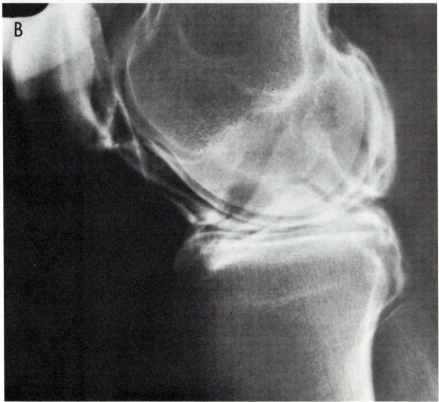

Popliteal Cyst—Baker's Cyst (cont.)

FIG 4–21 (cont.).

Typical

C, A popliteal cyst is a distended gastrocnemio-
semimembranous bursa that communicates with
the posterior portion of the knee joint through a
small channel and is usually identified with knee
in flexion. The cyst is medial and posterior.

Rupture of Popliteal Cyst

D, E, Arthrographic demonstration of contrast
leaking into the soft tissues with a feathery contour posterior to the popliteal cyst. *(Continued.)*

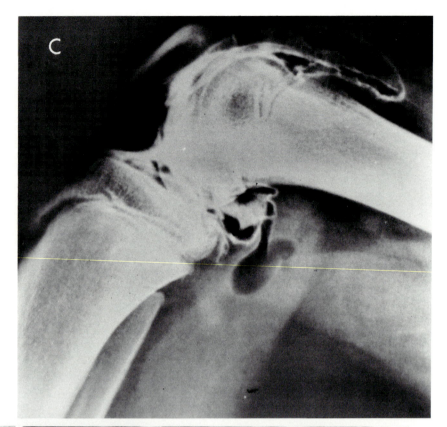

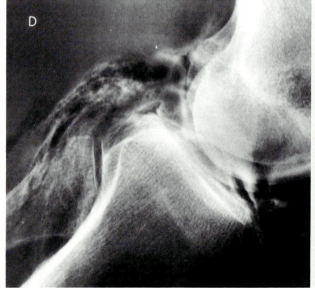

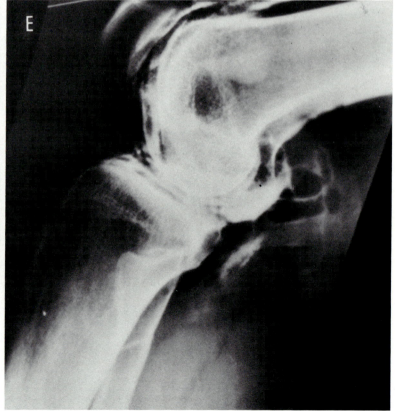

Dissection of Popliteal Cyst

FIG 4–21 (cont.).
F, Inferior extension of the popliteal cyst down the calf. The contrast remains contained by the cyst. (Permission for **D, F** granted courtesy of Pavlov H, Schneider R: Extrameniscal abnormalities as diagnosed by knee arthrography. *Radiol Clin North Am* 1981; 19:287.)

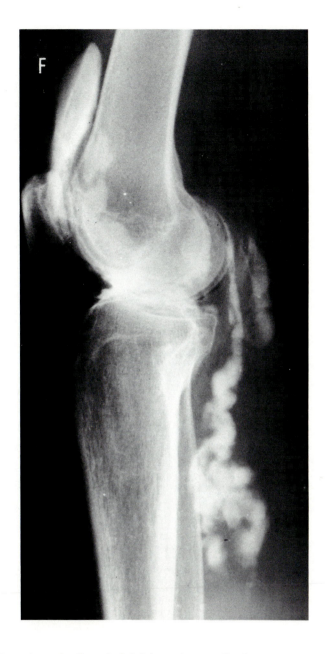

Popliteal Cyst—Baker's Cyst

REMEDY

Cyst with or without rupture: in the skeletal immature patient: treatment of a popliteal cyst is expectant observation since a popliteal cyst usually disappears. In the skeletal mature or pre-middle-age knee: for a Baker's cyst associated with intra-articular pathology (i.e., meniscal derangements), surgical treatment is directed toward intra-articular pathology.
Dissection: evaluate for intra-articular pathology and/or rheumatoid disorders.

Tibial-Fibular Capsular Recess

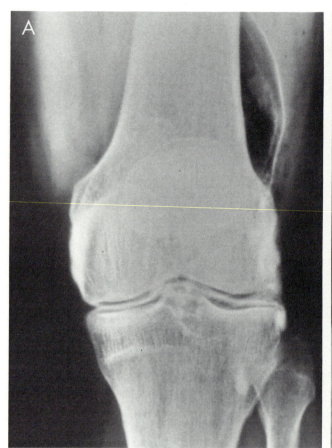

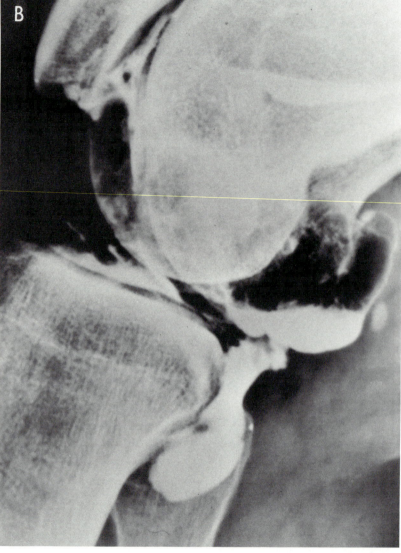

Normal

FIG 4–22.
A, B (both same patient), Capsular extension into the tibial-fibular recess can be distinguished from a popliteal cyst by its lateral location. It can be a site for loose bodies to collect.

Tibial-Fibular Capsular Recess

REMEDY   None, unless there are loose bodies collected in the recess that require surgical removal.

NONOSSEOUS INJURIES

Patellar Tendon

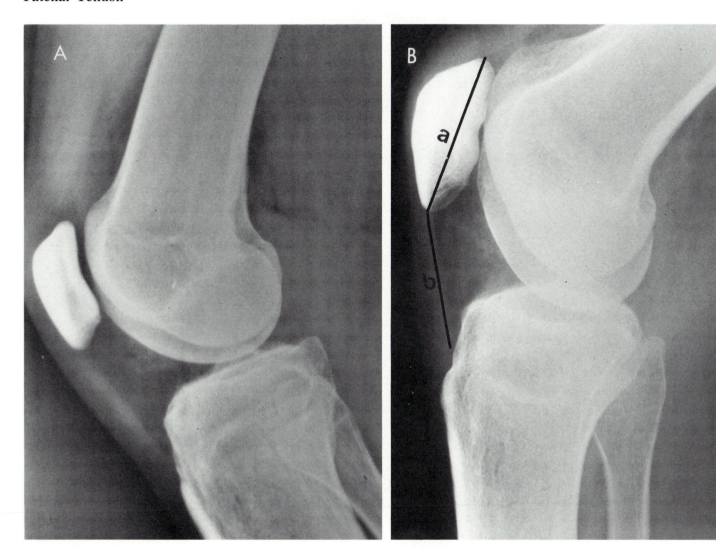

Normal

FIG 4–23.
A, The normal patellar tendon is well-defined posteriorly and the AP dimension is between 4 and 9 mm.
B, The patella to patellar tendon ratio *(a:b)* is approximately 1:1.2 (Ref: Insall J, Salvati E: Patella position in the normal knee joint. *Radiology* 1971; 101:101–104.) *(Continued.)*

Patellar Tendon

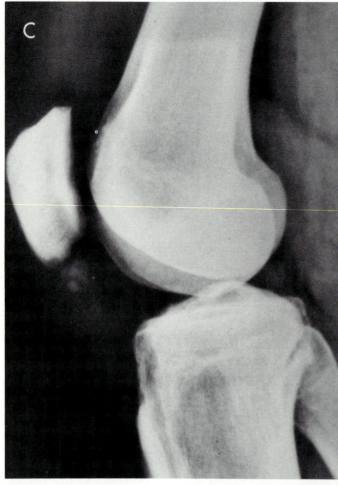

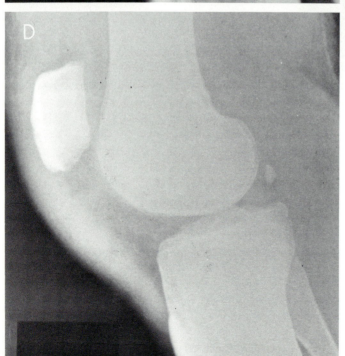

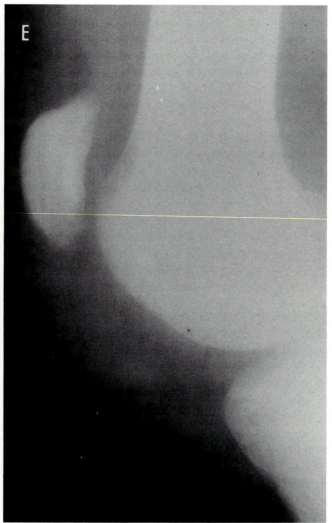

Ossicle in Patellar Tendon

FIG 4–23 (cont.).
C, Single or multiple ossicles within the patellar tendon at its insertion on the inferior pole of the patella may be a normal variant or symptomatic.

Rupture of Patellar Tendon

D, E, Lateral views of knees in two patients. Radiograph is as obtained using a soft-tissue technique (low kV) and demonstrates a patellar tendon rupture. The patellar tendon is thick and poorly defined and the patella is too high. *(Continued.)*

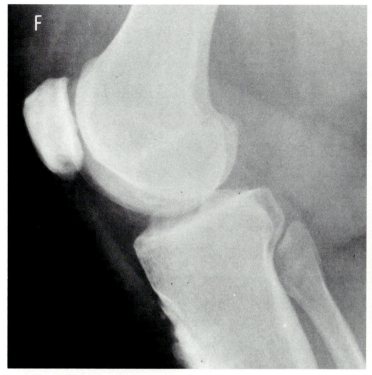 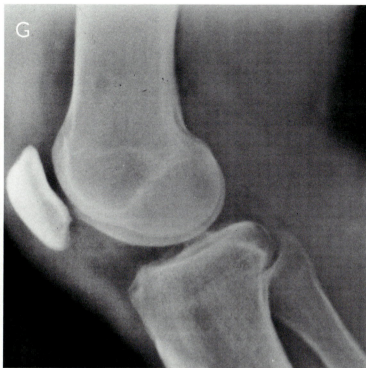

Avulsion of Patellar Tendon

FIG 4–23 (cont.).
F, The patellar tendon is of normal thickness and is well-delineated posteriorly but the radiolucency at its insertion point into the inferior pole of the patellar indicates avulsion. The patella to patellar tendon ratio is abnormal and the patella is superiorly displaced.

Tendonitis—Patellar Tendon

G, The posterior aspect of the patellar tendon is thick and poorly defined proximally at its origin on the patella.

Patellar Tendon

REMEDY

Ossicle: if symptomatic, surgical removal.
Rupture or avulsion: surgical repair.
Tendinitis: isometric exercise, ice, and oral systemic anti-inflammatory agents.

Osgood Schlatter Disease

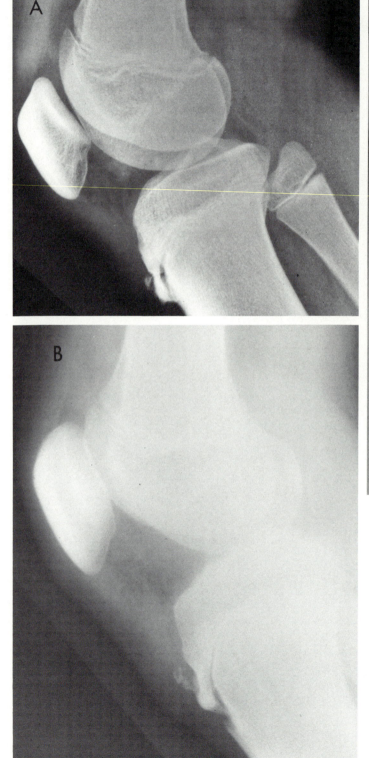

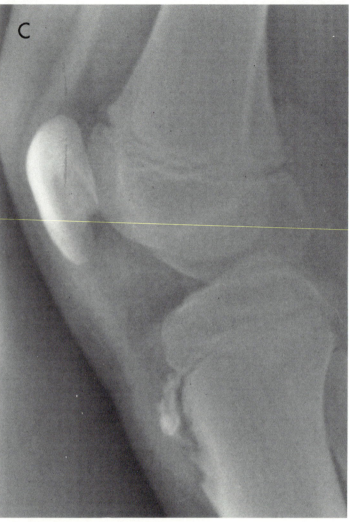

FIG 4–24.
A–C, Three examples that demonstrate the three radiographic signs that must be associated with clinical symptoms: (1) thickening and irregularity of the patellar tendon; (2) soft-tissue swelling anterior to the tibial tubercle; and (3) fragmentation and irregularity of the tibial tubercle. (Permission for **A** granted courtesy of Insall JN: *Surgery of the Knee.* New York, Churchill Livingstone, 1984.) *(Continued.)*

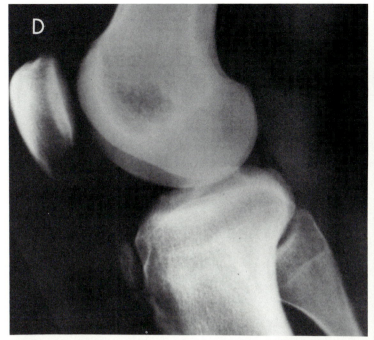

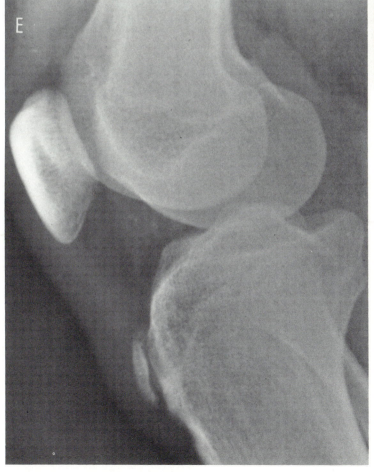

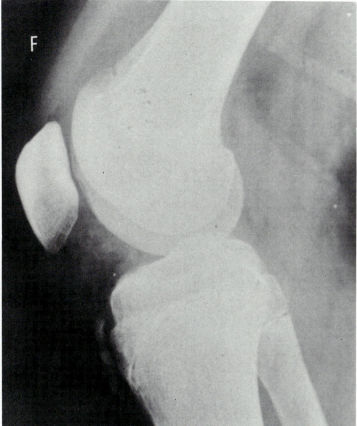

FIG 4–24 (cont.).
D–F, Three examples of an intratendinous ossicle secondary to failure of the apophysis to unite with the tibia. This is usually identified in the older patient after the epiphysis has fused.

Remedy appears on the following page.

Osgood Schlatter Disease

REMEDY

Treatment depends on clinical and roentgenographic findings. *Insertional tendinitis* (possible normal x-rays) and/or *fragmentation* and *irregularity* of the tibial tubercle: treat conservatively with decreased activity.

With the presence of a *separate residual ossicle* at the tibial tubercle, usually seen in the mature skeleton: surgical excision, if symptomatic.

Medial Collateral Ligament Rupture

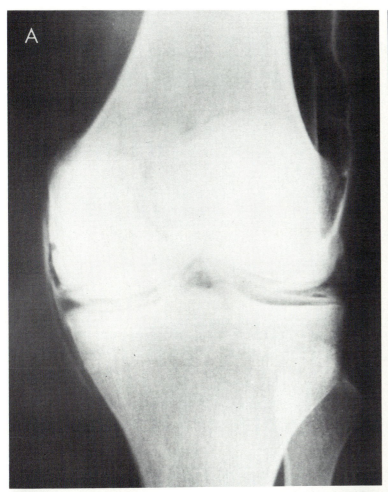

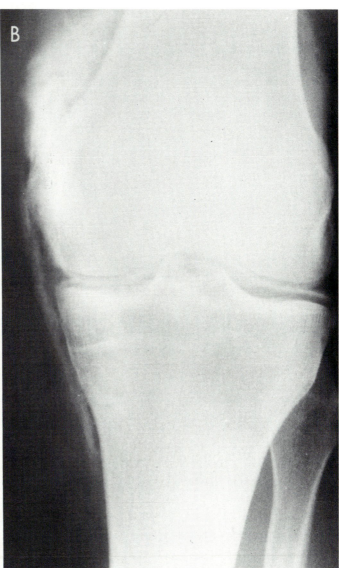

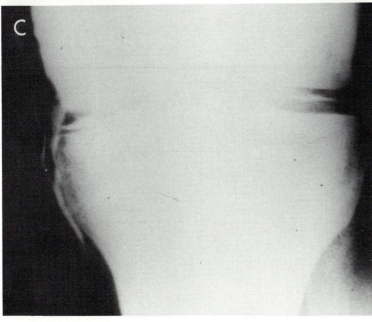

Acute Injury

FIG 4–26.
A–C, Three examples of acute tears of the deep layer
of the medial collateral ligament, demonstrated by arthrography. The smooth peripheral border to the ex-
travasated contrast indicates that the superficial portion of the medial collateral ligament is intact.
(Permission for **B** granted courtesy of Pavlov H: Sports
related knee injuries, in Taveras JM (ed): *Radiology/
Diagnosis/Imaging/Intervention.* Philadelphia, JB Lippincott Co, 1986.) *(Continued.)*

Medial Collateral Ligament Rupture—Acute Injury (cont.)

FIG 4–26 (cont.).
D, An example of an acute tear of the deep and superficial layers of the medial collateral ligament. A feathery appearance of the contrast within the medial soft tissues indicates a tear of the deep and superficial layers of the medial collateral ligament. *(Continued.)*

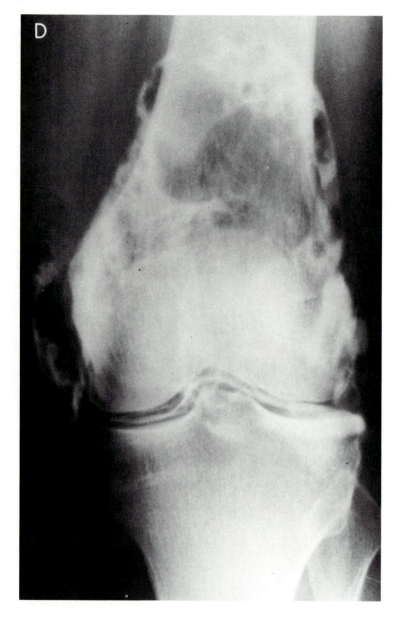

FIG 4–26 (cont.).
E, Increased distance between the tibia and the femur during arthrography indicates medial collateral ligament laxity; the contrast present in the adjacent soft tissues indicates the ligament is torn and the tear is acute. (Permission for **C, E** granted courtesy of Pavlov H, Schneider R: Extrameniscal abnormalities as diagnosed by knee arthrography. *Radiol Clin North Am* 1981; 19:287.)

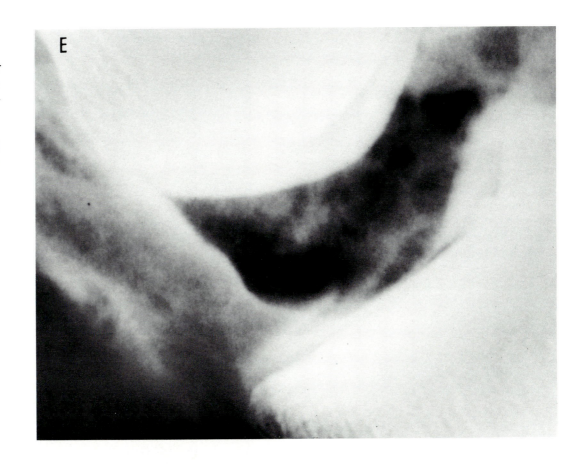

Medial Collateral Ligament Rupture—Acute Injury

REMEDY

Isolated acute tear: conservative treatment.
Acute tear combined with torn anterior cruciate ligament: both ligaments should be surgically repaired.

Medial Collateral Ligament Rupture (cont.)

Chronic Injury—Pellegrini-Steida Disease

Pellegrini Steida disease is calcification and/or ossification within the medial collateral ligament secondary to a previous injury. The ossification results from an intraligamentous hemorrhage that subsequently calcifies and ossifies.

FIG 4–27.
A, Calcification at the origin of the medial collateral ligament. **B, C,** Two examples of calcification within the substance of the ligament. (**C** *appears on facing page.*) (Permission for **A, B** granted courtesy of Insall JN: Surgery of the Knee. New York, Churchill Livingstone, 1984.)

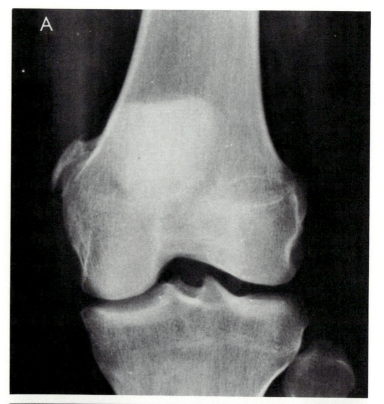

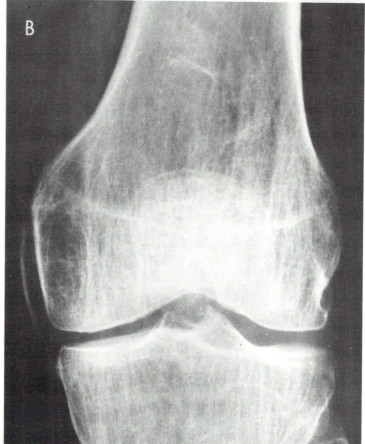

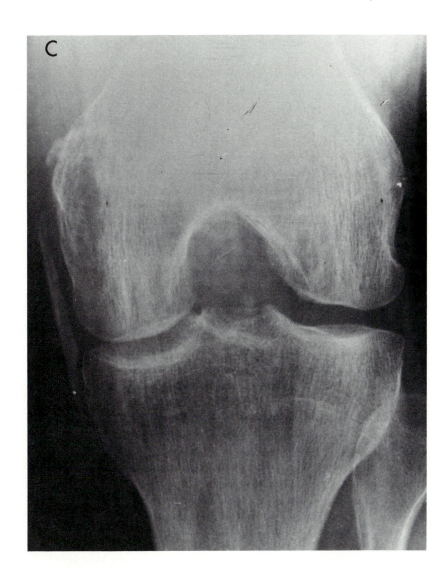

Medial Collateral Ligament Rupture
Chronic Injury—Pellegrini-Steida Disease

REMEDY This is primarily a radiographic finding indicative of an old injury; no treatment is necessary.

Lateral Capsular Ligament Rupture

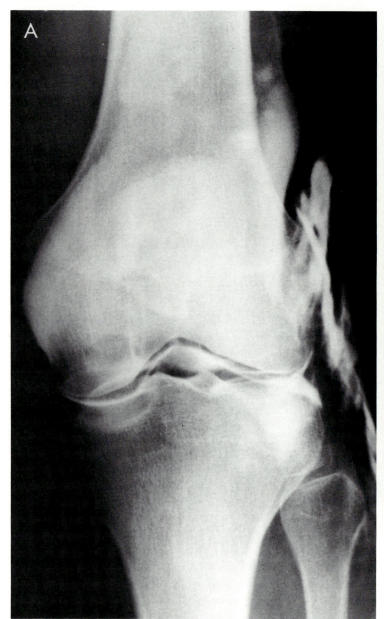

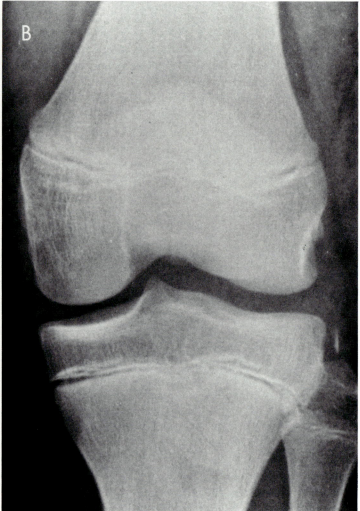

FIG 4–28.
A, Arthrographic demonstration of a tear of the
lateral capsular ligament with contrast leaking
through the meniscal capsular (the intra-articular)
portion. (Permission for **A** granted courtesy of
Pavlov H, Schneider R: Extrameniscal abnormalities as diagnosed by knee arthrography. *Radiol
Clin North Am* 1981; 19:287.) *(Continued.)*

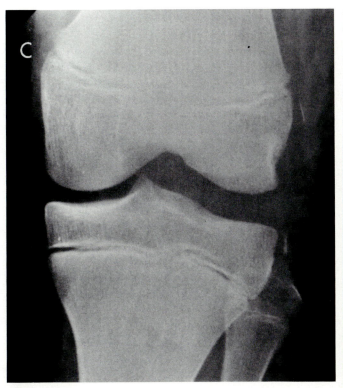

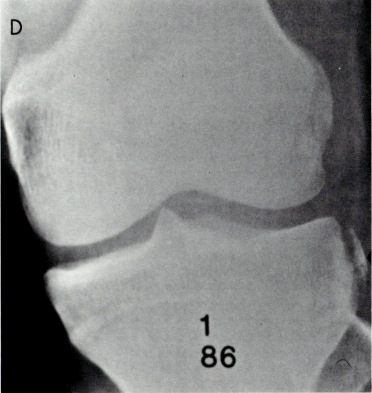

FIG 4–28 (cont.).
B–E, Four examples of a "capsular sign" or a Segond fracture: the sliver of bone adjacent to the lateral tibial plateau indicates an avulsion of the inferior meniscal capsular attachment. (**E** *appears on the following page.*) (Ref: Segond, P: Recherches cliniques et experimentales, Sur les epanchements sanguins du genou par entorse. *Prog Med* 7:297, 319, 340, 379, 400, 419, 879.) (*Continued.*)

Lateral Capsular Ligament Rupture (cont.)

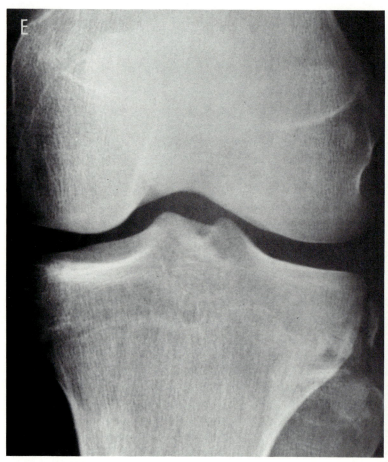

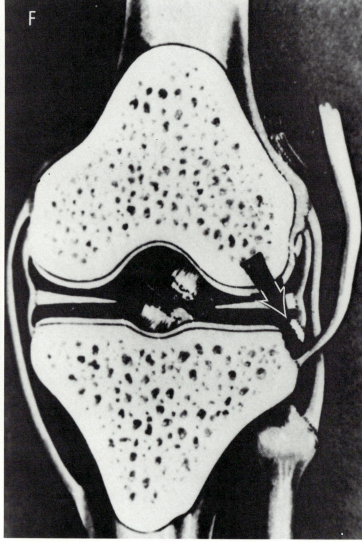

FIG 4–28 (cont.).
F, This injury, a Segond fracture or a "capsular sign" *(arrow),* is significant because of a high incidence of an associated anterior cruciate ligament injury. (Permission for **F** granted courtesy of Woods GW, Stanley RF, Tullos HS: Lateral capsular sign: X-ray clue to a significant knee instability. *Am J Sports Med* 1979; 7:27.)

Lateral Capsular Ligament Rupture

REMEDY   Surgical repair and/or reconstruction of anterior cruciate ligament.

FEMUR

Normal Variants

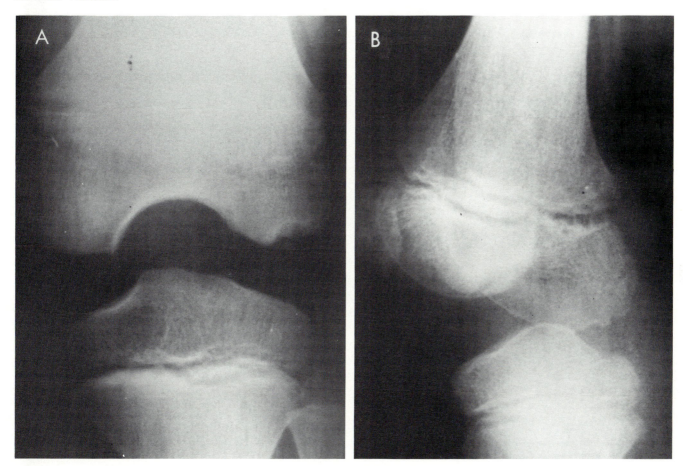

FIG 4–29.
A–C (**A, B** are same patient), Irregularity of the posterior surface of either or both femoral condyles simulates osteochondritis dissecans. However, this is a *normal variant*, commonly identified in 8- to 10-year-old children, and is of no clinical significance. Because this finding occurs on the posterior surface of the condyles it is best seen on the notch or tunnel view. (Permission granted courtesy of Insall JN: *Surgery of the Knee*. New York, Churchill Livingstone, 1984.) (*Note:* **C** *appears on following page.*)

Normal Variant (cont.)

FIG 4–29 (cont.).

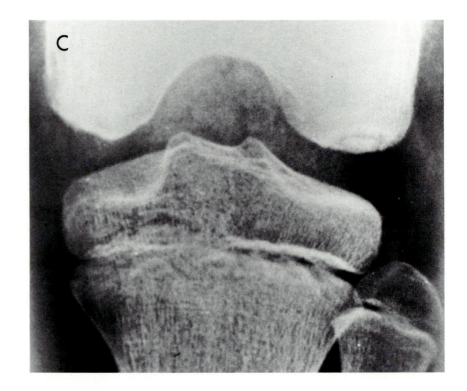

Normal Variant

REMEDY   None.

Osteochondritis Dissecans/Osteochondral Fracture

There are various radiographic patterns and femoral locations of these lesions. The patterns are sclerotic, lytic, or mixed. The sclerotic form is associated with a mature osseous body; the lytic pattern is associated with a fibrocartilaginous body; and the mixed pattern is associated with an osteochondral body. Arthrography is helpful to demonstrate the pattern of the articular cartilage overlying the osseous defect. Examples appear on the following pages.

Osteochondritis Dissecans/Osteochondral Fracture (cont.)

FIG 4–30.
A–C (all same patient), Osteochondritis dissecans is typically located on the intercondylar aspect of the medial femoral condyle and the lesion can usually be identified on the routine AP view in addition to the lateral and tunnel views. This is an example of the sclerotic form. The patient is skeletally mature. (*Continued.*)

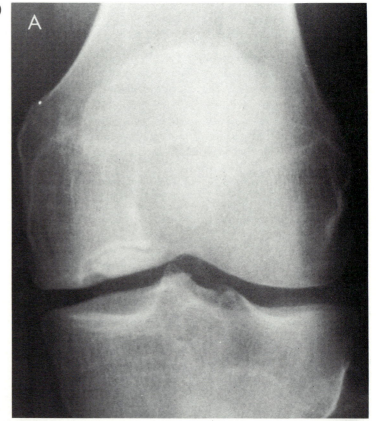

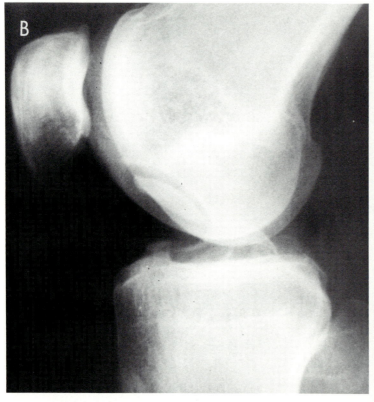

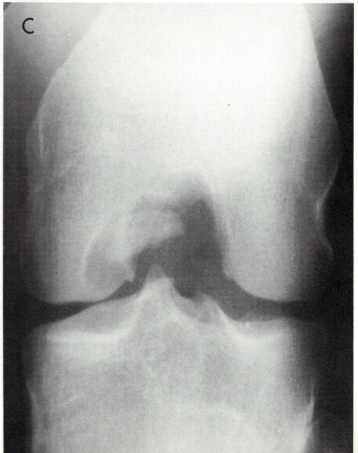

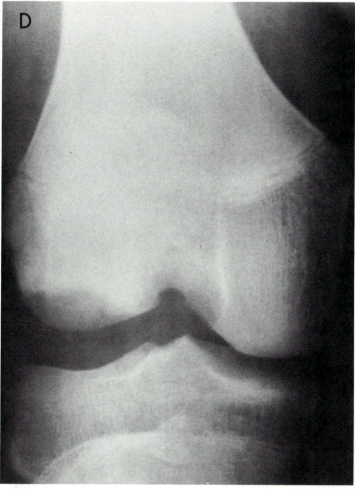

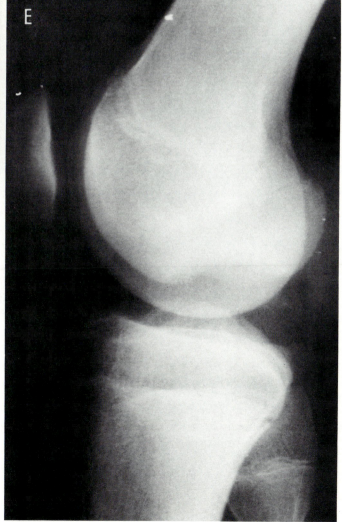

FIG 4–30 (cont.).
D, E (both same patient), AP and lateral views demonstrate the lytic form of osteochondritis dissecans or an osteochondral fracture in the lateral femoral condyle. Note the sclerotic base to the lesion. An arthrogram would be helpful to confirm a cartilaginous or loose body within the osseous defect. The epiphysis are open. (*Continued.*)

Osteochondritis Dissecans/Osteochondral Fracture (cont.)

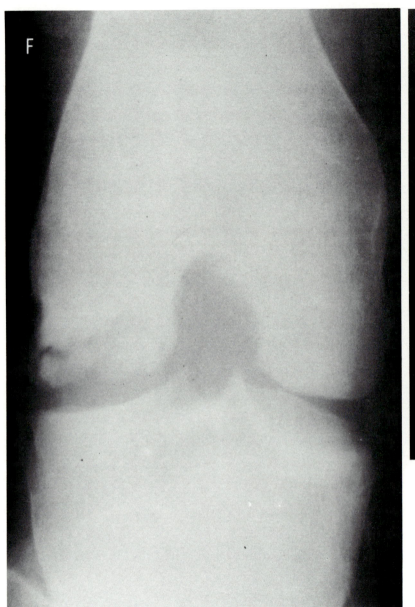
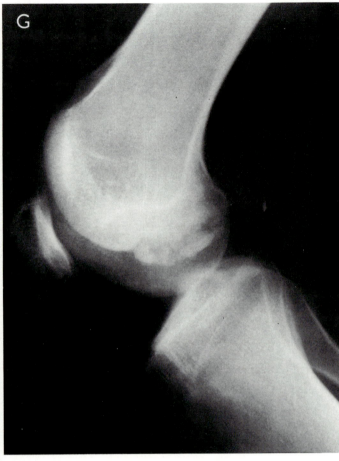

FIG 4–30 (cont.).
F, G (both same patient), AP and lateral views
demonstrate the mixed pattern of an osteochondritis dissecans or an osteochondral fracture in a
skeletally mature patient. (Permission for **B–E, G**
granted courtesy of Insall JN: *Surgery of the
Knee.* New York, Churchill Livingstone, 1984.)
(*Continued.*)

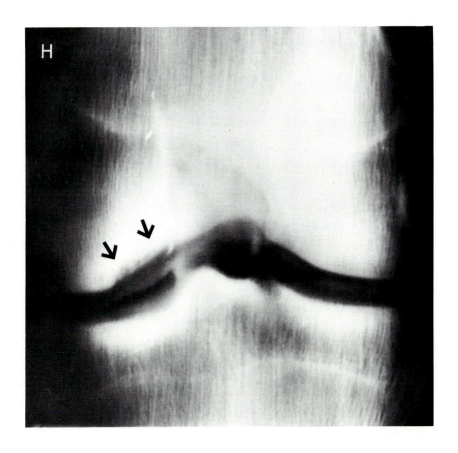

FIG 4–30 (cont.).
H, arthrotomogram demonstrates an intact articular cartilage over a mixed pattern of osteochondritis dissecans. The base of the osseous lesion is sclerotic *(arrows)*.

Osteochondritis Dissecans/Osteochondral Fracture (cont.)

FIG 4–30 (cont.).
I, An arthrogram demonstrates a notched articular cartilage defect that conforms to the lytic defect on the weight-bearing aspect of the condyle. An osteochondral fragment is probably loose within the joint. (Permission for **H** granted courtesy of Pavlov H, Schneider R: Extrameniscal abnormalities as diagnosed by knee arthrography. *Radiol Clin North Am* 1981; 19:287.)

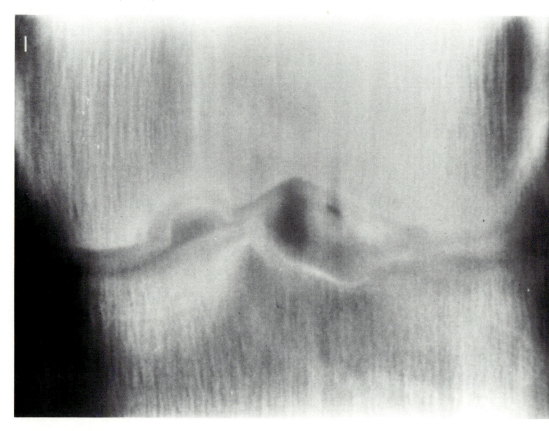

Osteochondritis Dissecans/Osteochondral Fracture

REMEDY

With objective findings, i.e., quadriceps atrophy and/or an effusion: an arthrogram and/or arthroscopy is recommended to determine the presence of an attached or loose cartilaginous fragment within the defect.

Without objective findings: careful observation is recommended.

In a skeletally immature patient: a loose fragment should be either removed or the base curetted and the fragment reattached.

In a skeletally mature patient: for small sclerotic osteochondritis dissecans lesion, i.e., smaller than its bed, excision is recommended. For large osteochondral lesions, treatment is aimed at surgical fixation to affect healing.

Lucent Articular Lesion in Lateral Femoral Condyle

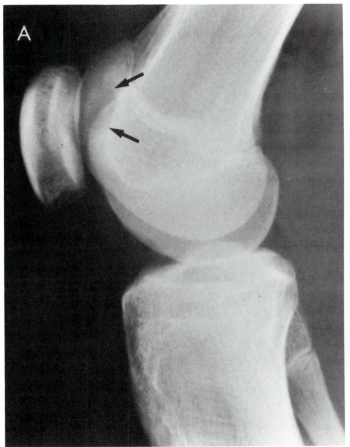
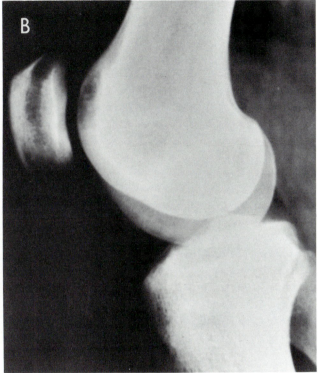

FIG 4–31.
A, B, Two examples: on the lateral view, an osteochondral fracture or osteochondritis dissecans is seen as a vague radiolucency *(arrows)* in the anterior aspect of the distal femoral epiphysis in the region of the patellar femoral joint. *(Continued.)*

Lucent Articular Lesion in Lateral Femoral Condyle (cont.)

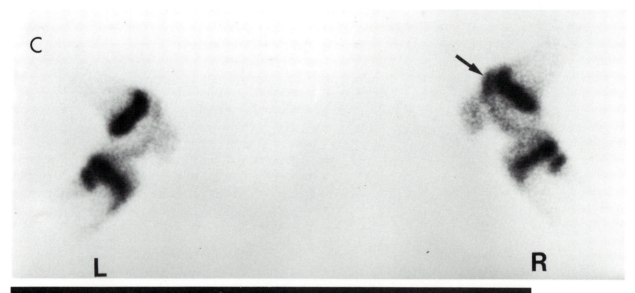

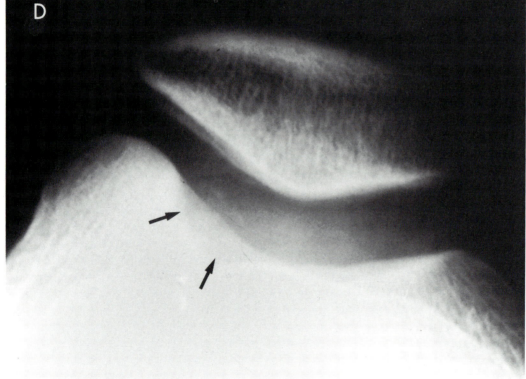

FIG 4–31 (cont.).
C, A radionuclide bone scan delineates augmented isotope uptake corresponding to this radiolucent lesion *(arrow).*
D–F, The Merchant view best demonstrates the lesion *(arrows).* The pattern of the lesion is similar to the description of osteochondritis dissecans/osteochondral fracture (see Fig 4–30) and can be mixed (**D**), lytic (**E**), or sclerotic (**F**). *(Continued.)*

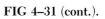

FIG 4–31 (cont.).

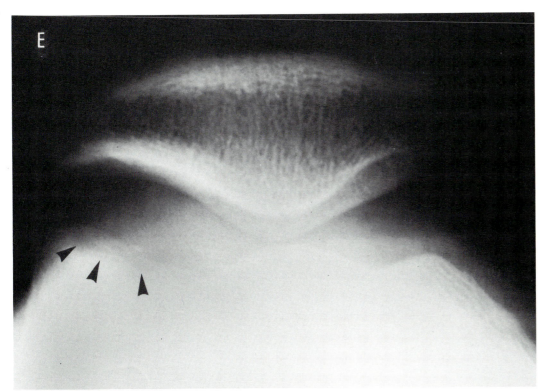

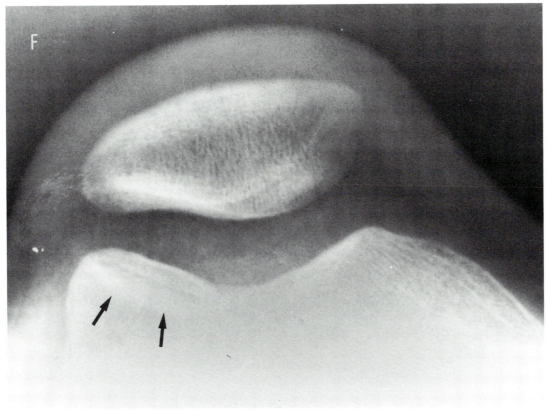

Lucent Articular Lesion in Lateral Femoral Condyle (cont.)

FIG–31 (cont.).
An arthrogram (**G,** same patient as **F**) demonstrates the articular cartilage over the sclerotic lesion in this patient to be intact. The Merchant view (described in Fig 4–10) demonstrates the femur at the patellar femoral joint, compared to the skyline view (**H**) performed with the knee in maximum flexion. On the skyline view, the patella is seen in tangent but the portion of the femur visualized is not that at the patellar femoral joint. (Permission for (**A–G**) granted courtesy of Cayea PD, Pavlov H, Sherman MF, et al: Lucent articular lesion in the lateral femoral condyle: A source of patellar femoral pain in the athletic adolescent. *AJR* 1981; 137:1145.)

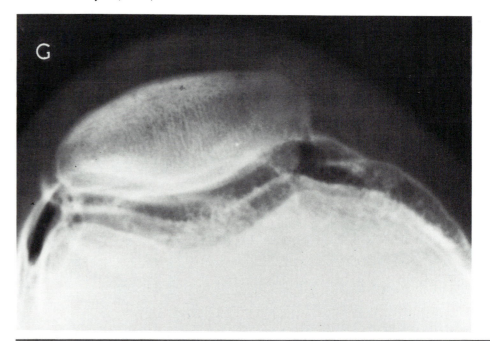

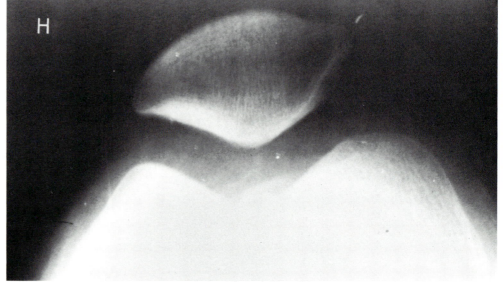

Lucent Articular Lesion in Lateral Femoral Condyle

REMEDY

Without objective findings: careful observation is recommended. *With objective findings,* i.e., quadriceps atrophy and/or an effusion: an arthrogram and/or arthroscopy is recommended to determine the presence of an attached or loose cartilage within the defect. Loose fragment should be either removed or the base curetted and the fragment reattached.

Transchondral Fracture

FIG 4–32.
A purely cartilaginous defect confined within the articular cartilage will be demonstrated only on arthrography or at arthroscopy. In this instance, the defect is in the weight bearing portion of the lateral femoral condyle. (Permission granted courtesy of Pavlov H, Schneider R: Extrameniscal abnormalities as diagnosed by knee arthrography. *Radio Clin North Am* 1981;19:287.)

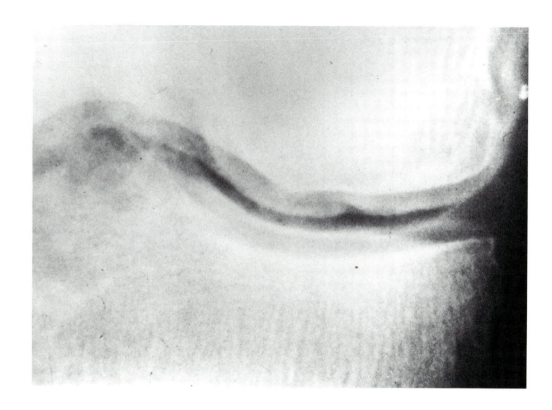

Transchondral Fracture

REMEDY   Arthroscopic removal of loose fragment.

CHAPTER 5

The Femur

INTERCONDYLAR

Salter III Fracture

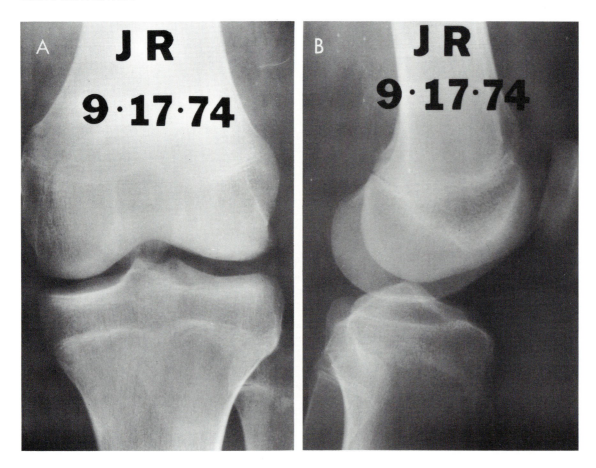

FIG 5–1.
A, B (A–D are all the same patient), AP and lateral views appear normal. *(Continued.)*

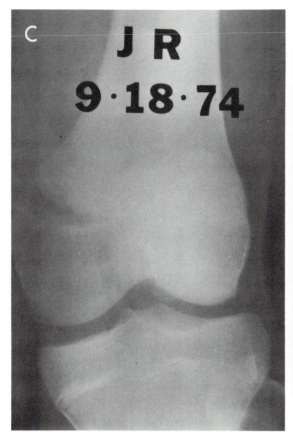

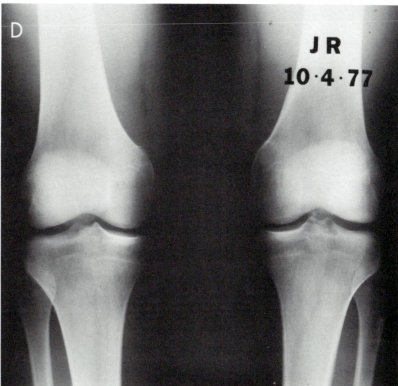

FIG 5–1 (cont.).
C, Stress views obtained under fluoroscopy demonstrate widening of the medial growth plate; however, stress views are not recommended as they can result in growth disturbances or articular surface irregularities and joint incongruity. **D,** The patient healed without growth disturbances. (*Continued.*)

Salter III Fracture (cont.)

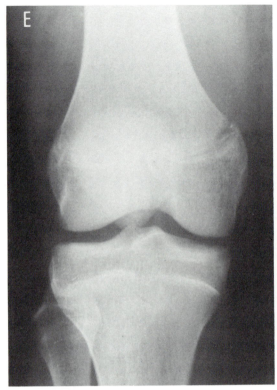

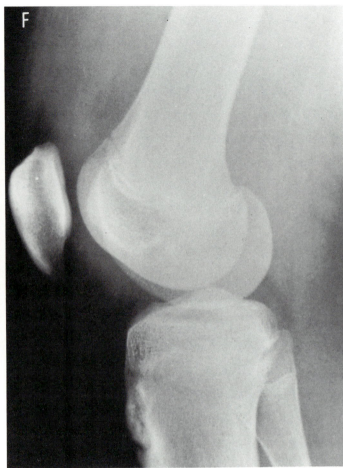

FIG 5–1 (cont.).
E–H (all same patient), Frontal view of the knee demonstrates widening of the medial growth plate; **F,** lateral view demonstrates a joint effusion, but the epiphyseal growth plate appears normal. *(Continued.)*

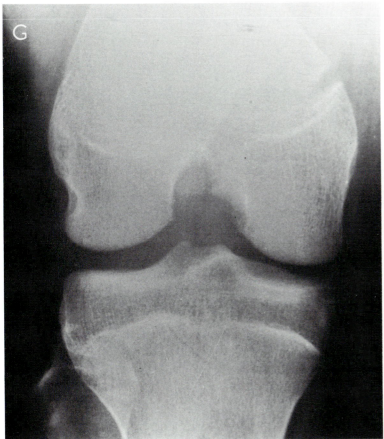

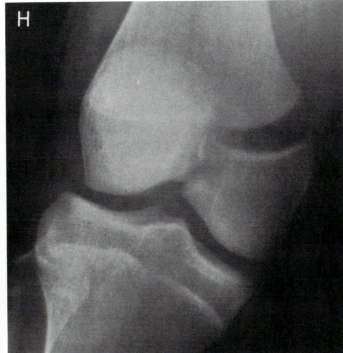

FIG 5–1 (cont.).
G, On the tunnel view, a vertical radiolucency in
the intercondylar notch is identified.
H, Valgus stress of the knee should be avoided
as the entire medial femoral condylar fragment
can become displaced. (*Continued.*)

Salter III Fracture (cont.)

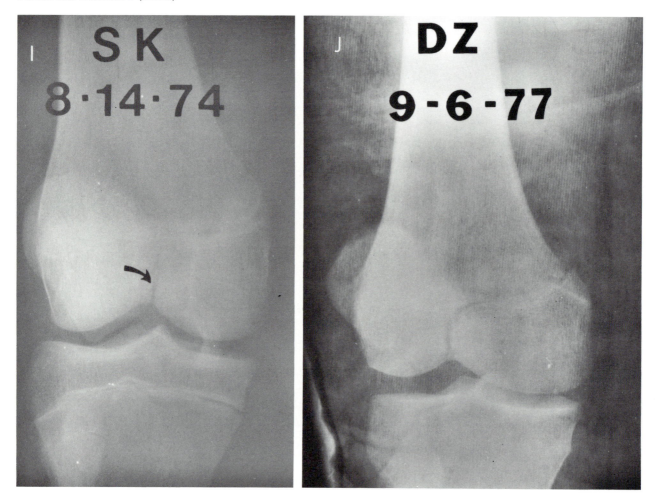

FIG 5–1 (cont.).
I, J, The oblique view of the knee (two examples) is the best view to identify the vertical fracture line *(arrow)*. *(Continued.)*

FIG 5–1 (cont.).
K (same patient as **J**), In some instances the horizontal component of the fracture is seen on the lateral view. (Permission for **A, B, C, I, J, K** granted courtesy of Torg JS, Pavlov H, Morris VB: Salter-Harris type III fracture of the medial femoral condyle occurring in the adolescent athlete. *J Bone Joint Surg* 1981; 63A:586.)

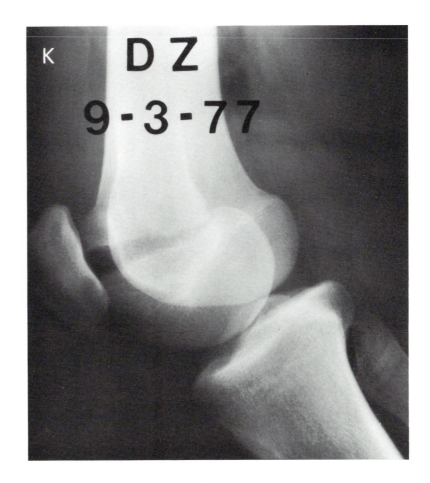

Salter III Fracture

REMEDY:

If *nondisplaced:* cast immobilization, non-weight-bearing on crutches.

If *displaced:* reduction.

Attention should be paid to disruption of the anterior cruciate ligament. The pathomechanics of a Salter-Harris type-III fracture of the medial femoral condyle involve a valgus force applied to the distal part of the femur and the knee, resulting in a fracture across the medial aspect of the distal femoral physis that extends through the epiphysis into the intercondylar notch **(a).** The medial condylar fragment is held in relation to the proximal part of the tibia by the medial collateral and posterior cruciate ligaments **(b).** The lateral femoral condylar fragment rotates on the lateral tibial condyle either laterally or posteriorly, or both. Because of the restraining effect of the anterior cruciate and lateral capsular ligaments, spontaneous reduction occurs **(c).** With excessive rotation of the femoral lateral condylar fragment, the anterior cruciate ligament becomes vulnerable to injury. (Permission for diagram granted courtesy of Torg JS, Pavlov H, Morris VB: Salter-Harris type III fracture of the medial femoral condyle occurring in the adolescent athlete. *J Bone Joint Surg* 1981; 63A:586.)

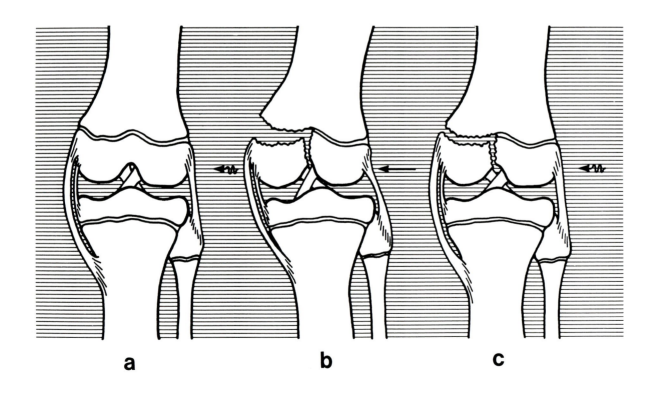

a   b   c

SUPRACONDYLAR

Stress Reaction and/or Fracture—Distal Femur

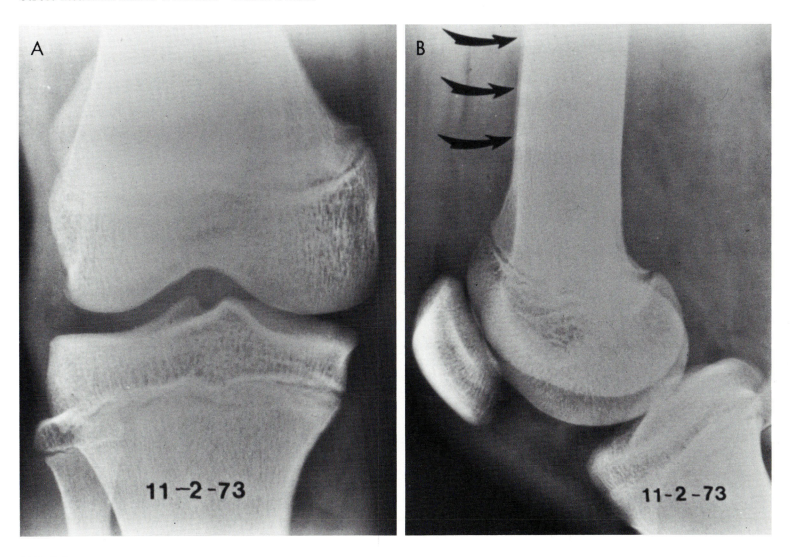

FIG 5–2.
A, B (both same patient), (11–2–73) Anteroposterior (AP) and lateral views demonstrate faint periosteal reactions anterior to distal femoral diaphysis on the lateral view *(arrows)*. This frontal view was coned to close to the supracondylar area and the periosteal reaction of the femoral shaft identified on the lateral view was not appreciated. *(Continued.)*

Stress Reaction and/or Fracture—Distal Femur (cont.)

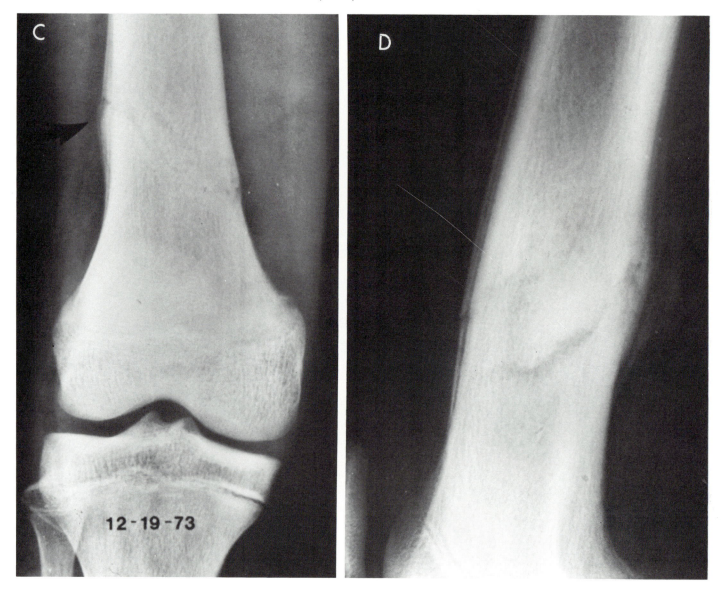

FIG 5–2 (cont.).
C, D, Three weeks later (12–19–73) AP and lateral views demonstrate periosteal new bone formation around the entire distal femoral shaft. The fracture line completely crosses the femoral shaft. *(Continued.)*

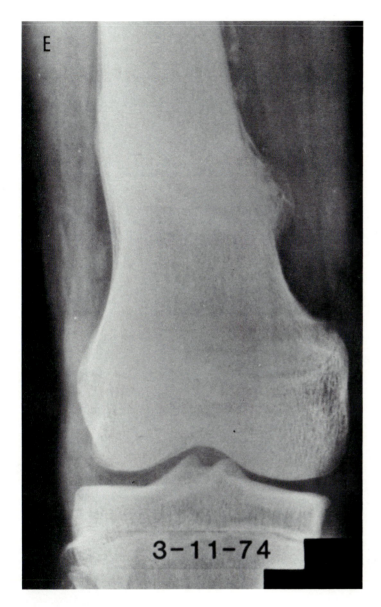

FIG 5–2 (cont.).
E, (3–11–74) Remodeling and healing is demonstrated. *(Continued.)*

Stress Reaction and/or Fracture—Distal Femur (cont.)

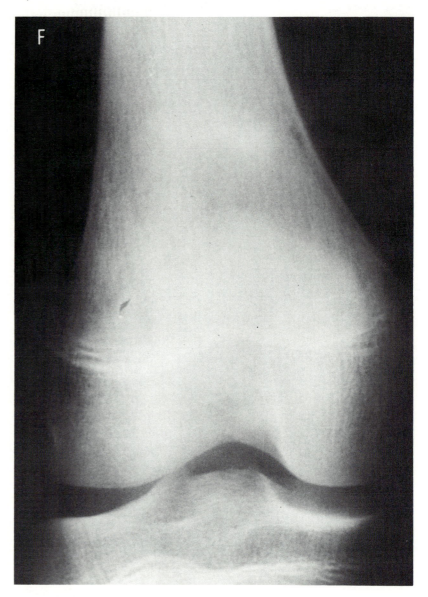

FIG 5–6 (cont.).
F–H (all same patient), Horizontal linear density in the distal femur at the metaphyseal-diaphyseal junction and periosteal new bone formation. A follow-up examination (**H**) demonstrates thickening of the periosteal new bone formation on the medial aspect of the distal femur.

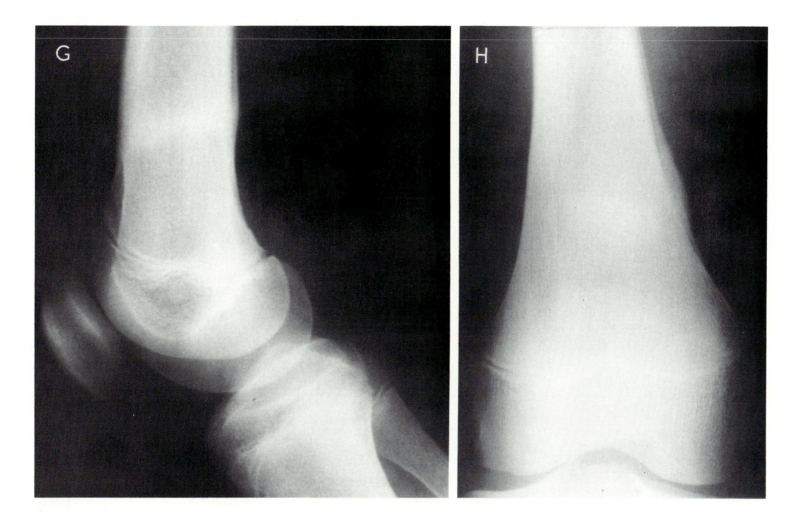

Stress Reaction and/or Fracture—Distal Femur

REMEDY

Incomplete diaphyseal stress fracture: non-weight-bearing on crutches.

Complete nondisplaced diaphyseal fracture: traction in acute phase and subsequent long leg cast immobilization.

OSTEOID OSTEOMA—FEMUR

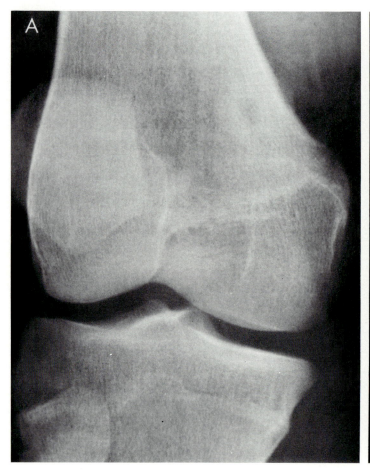

FIG 5–3.
A, Ovoid lucent nidus within an area of sclerosis is present in the medial supracondylar area.

B, Ovoid lucent nidus is demonstrated on a tomogram in the lateral supracondylar area *(arrow).* (Permission for **A, B** granted courtesy of Torg JS, Loughran T, Pavlov H, et al: Osteoid osteoma: Distant, periarticular and subarticular lesions as a cause of knee pain. *Sports Med* 1985; 2:296.)

Osteoid Osteoma—Femur

REMEDY: Surgical excision.

FEMORAL SHAFT

Stress Reaction and/or Fracture

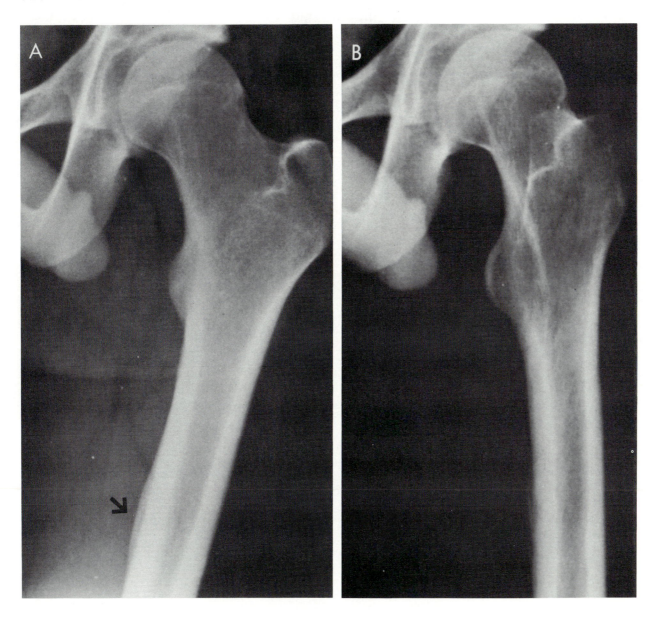

FIG 5–4.
A, B (both same patient), Frontal views of the femur obtained in internal and external rotation demonstrate periosteal and endosteal thickening of the medial cortex of the femoral diaphysis *(arrow)*. A definite fracture is not seen.

Stress Reaction and/or Fracture—Femoral Shaft

REMEDY   Activity limitation.

Osteoid Osteoma

FIG 5–5.
A,B (both same patient), The frontal view demonstrates increased density in the region of the lesser trochanter.

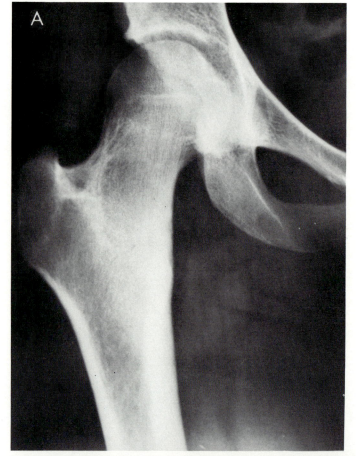

B, computed tomogram (CT) scan demonstrates the radiolucent nidus and the thickened sclerotic posterior femoral cortex. *(Continued.)*

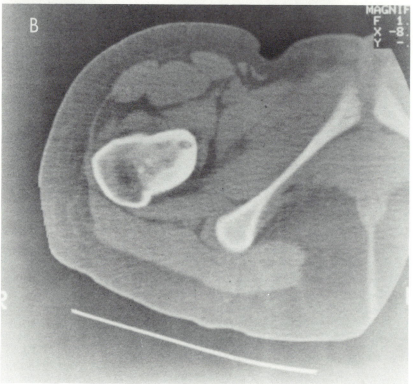

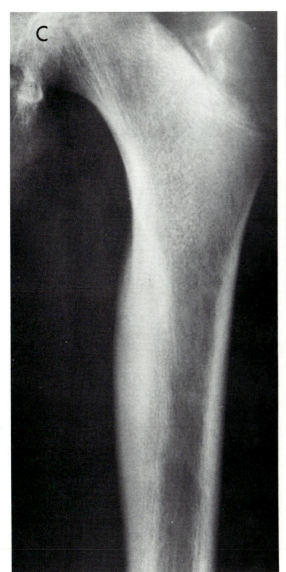

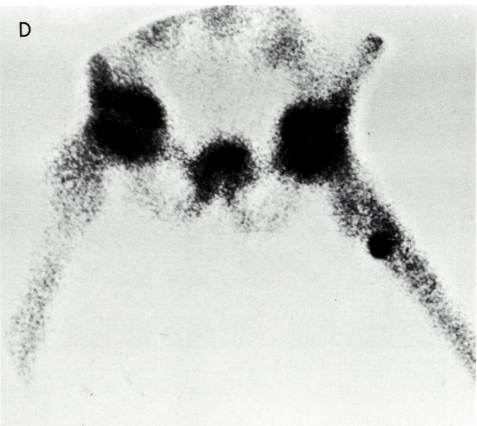

FIG 5–5 (cont.).
C,D (both same patient), The frontal view demonstrates an elongated area of cortical thickening along the medial aspect of the femoral shaft. **D,** Bone scan demonstrates the localized area of augmented isotope uptake consistent with an osteoid osteoma. (Permission for **A–D** granted courtesy of Torg JS, Loughran T, Pavlov H, et al: Osteoid osteoma: Distant, periarticular and subarticular lesions as a cause of knee pain. *Sports Med* 1985; 2:296.) *(Continued.)*

Osteoid Osteoma—Femoral Shaft (cont.)

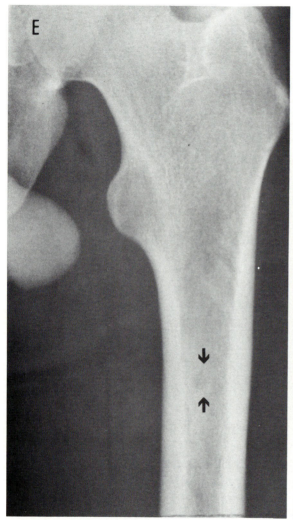

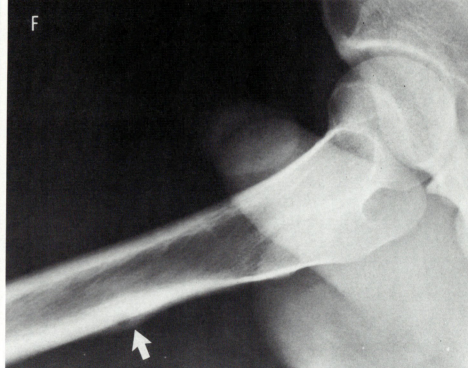

FIG 5–5 (cont.).
E,F (both same patient), Frontal and frog-leg lateral views demonstrate an ovoid lucency in the posterior cortex representing an osteoid osteoma (*arrows*).

Osteoid Osteoma—Femoral Shaft

REMEDY: Surgical excision.

PROXIMAL FEMUR, HIP

Stress Reaction and/or Fracture—Femur

Radionuclide Bone Scan

FIG 5–6.
A, B, C, Three examples in which there is localized augmented isotope uptake in the femoral neck on the left (**A, B**) in two patients, and on the right (**C**) in the other. In all instances, the radiographs were normal. (Note: **C** appears on following page.) (*Continued.*)

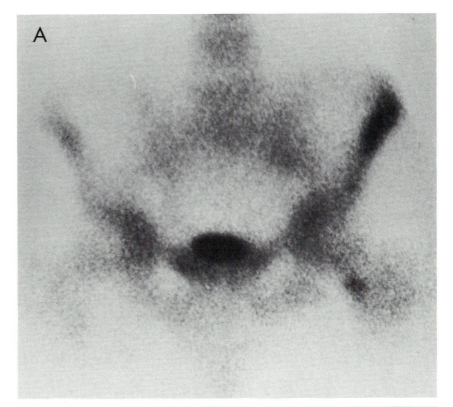

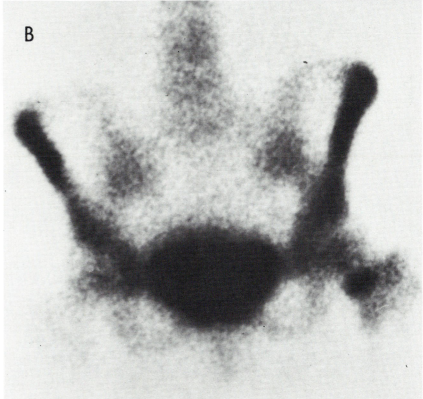

Stress Reaction and/or Fracture—Proximal Femur (cont.)

FIG 5–6 (cont.).

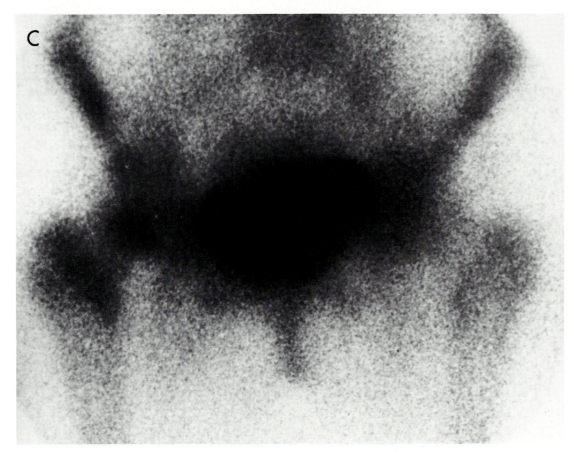

Typical Radiographic Scenarios

FIG 5–6 (cont.).
D,E (both same patient), Initial radiograph demonstrates normal findings, although there is a vague area of radiodensity just proximal to the lesser trochanter.

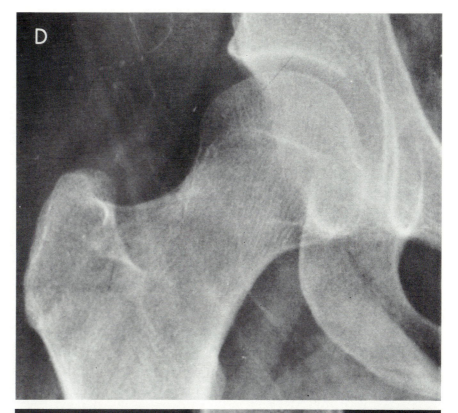

E, On a follow-up radiograph 3 weeks later, a definitive radiodense horizontal stress fracture *(arrow)* is identified in this region of the medial femoral neck, proximal to the lesser trochanter. *(Continued.)*

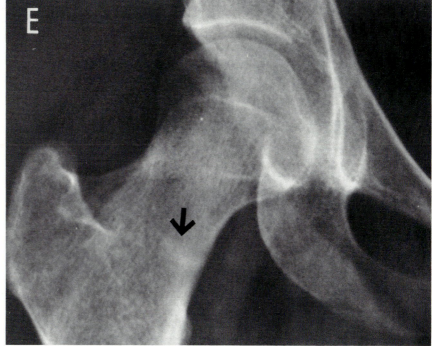

Stress Reaction and/or Fracture—Proximal Femur (cont.)

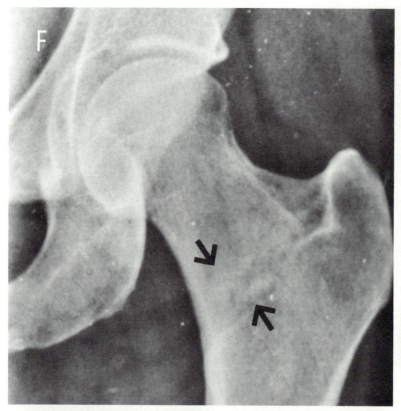

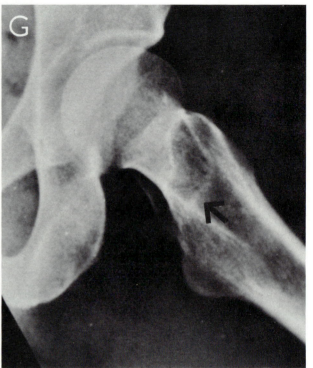

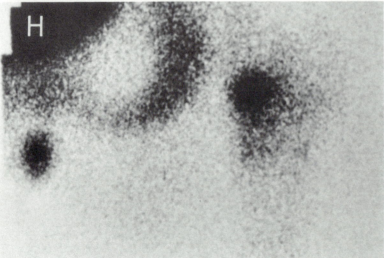

FIG 5–6 (cont.).
F–H (all same patient), Frontal and frog-leg lateral views demonstrate a vague horizontal area of increased density in the femoral neck, just proximal to the lesser trochanter *(arrows)*. **H,** On the bone scan, intense isotope augmentation is noted confirming this is a stress fracture of the hip. *(Continued.)*

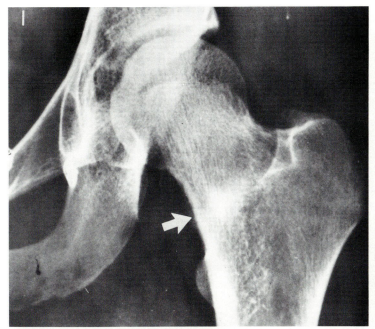

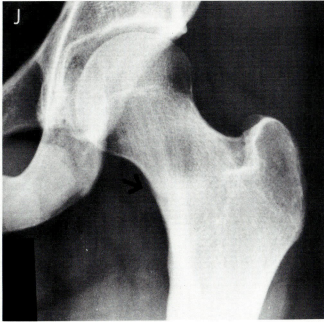

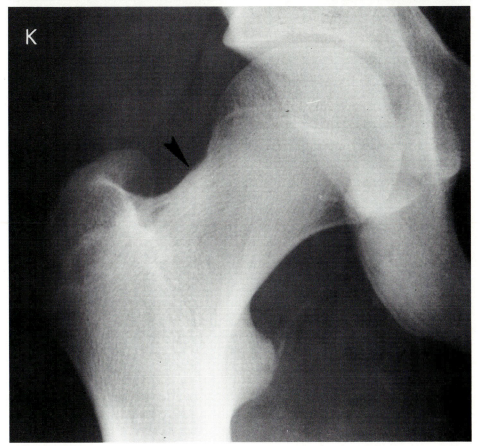

Varying Patterns of Femoral Neck Stress Fractures

FIG 5–6 (cont.).
I,J (both same patient), Initial radiograph demonstrates a wide radiodense zone *(arrow)* in the medial aspect of the femoral neck. **J,** Subsequent radiograph 10 days later demonstrates the radiolucent fracture *(arrow)* within the sclerotic area.

K, Radiodensity of the superolateral aspect of the femoral neck *(arrowhead)*. *(Continued.)*

Stress Reaction and/or Fracture (cont.)

*Varying Patterns of Femoral Neck Stress
Fractures (cont.)*

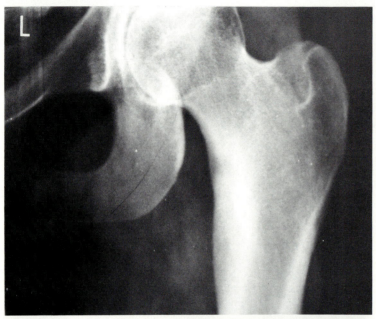

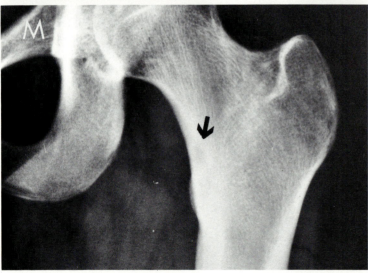

FIG 5–6 (cont.).
L,M (both same patient), Frontal view of the proximal femur in internal rotation demonstrates cortical thickening distal to the lesser trochanter.

M, In slightly increased external rotation, a circular radiolucency is identified just proximal to the lesser trochanter *(arrow)* and is indistinguishable from an osteoid osteoma. Clinical correlation is necessary for further evaluation and biopsy may be necessary for definitive evaluation. This patient responded to rest and the lucency represented a stress fracture. *(Continued.)*

FIG 5–6 (cont.).
N, Interruption of the medial cortex *(arrow)*.

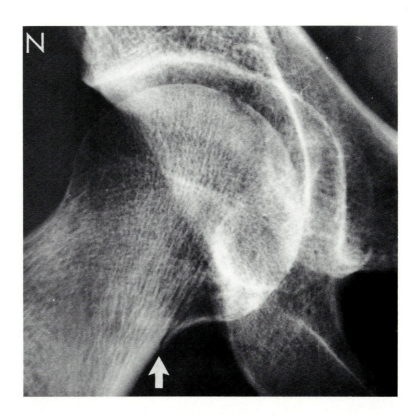

Stress Reaction and/or Fracture

REMEDY: *One cortex involvement:* non-weight-bearing, crutches, and close observation until healed.
Complete, nondisplaced fracture: internal fixation in situ.
Complete displaced fracture: open reduction and internal fixation is indicated.

Pseudo Fracture

FIG 5–7.
A, A circumferential osteophyte around the femoral neck can simulate an area of sclerosis and fracture *(arrow)* on the frog-leg lateral view.

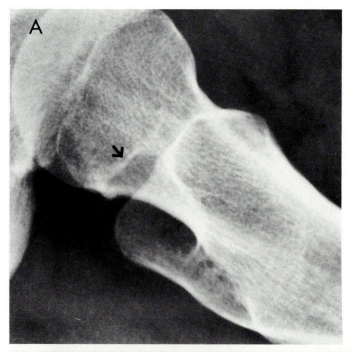

B (same patient as **A**), On the groin lateral view, the osteophyte around the femoral head is identified. The density on the frog-leg lateral can be distinguished from a stress fracture because the horizontal density is subcapital compared to the typical stress fracture that is intertrochanteric. (Compare figure to 5–6, **G**, page 270.)

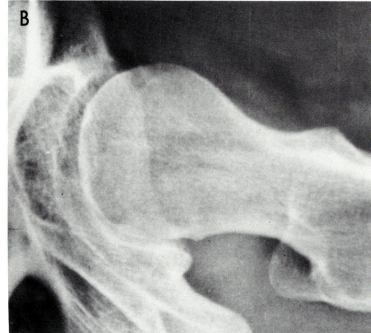

Pseudo Fracture

REMEDY   None.

SOFT-TISSUE INJURIES

Myositis Ossificans

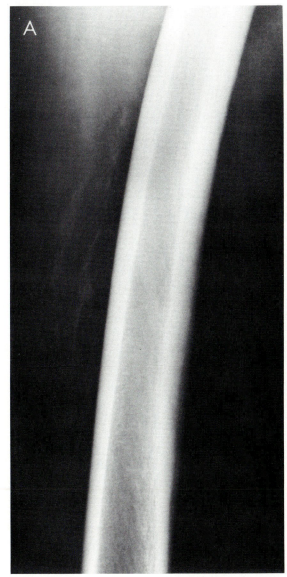

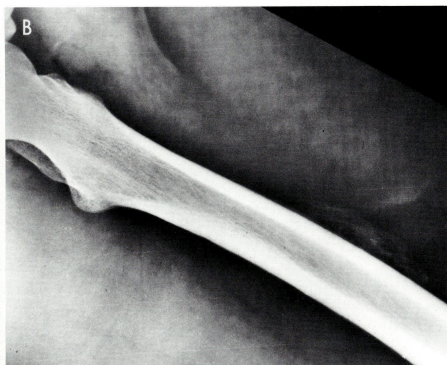

FIG 5–8.
A, B, C, D, Four examples of myositis ossification. Myositis ossificans occurs secondary to a previous hematoma within the muscle and occurs characteristically in the quadriceps tendon. The calcification is oriented along the long axis of the femoral shaft and is peripherally denser than centrally. (Note: **C, D** appear on following page.) (Ref: Norman A, Dorfman H: Juxta-cortical circumscribed myositis ossificans evaluation and radiologic features. *Radiology* 1970; 96:301–306.)

Myositis Ossificans (cont.)

FIG 5–8. (cont.).
(Permission for **A–D** granted courtesy of Pavlov H, Torg JS, Hersh A, et al: The roentgen examination of runners' injuries. *RadioGraphics* 1981; 1:17–34.)

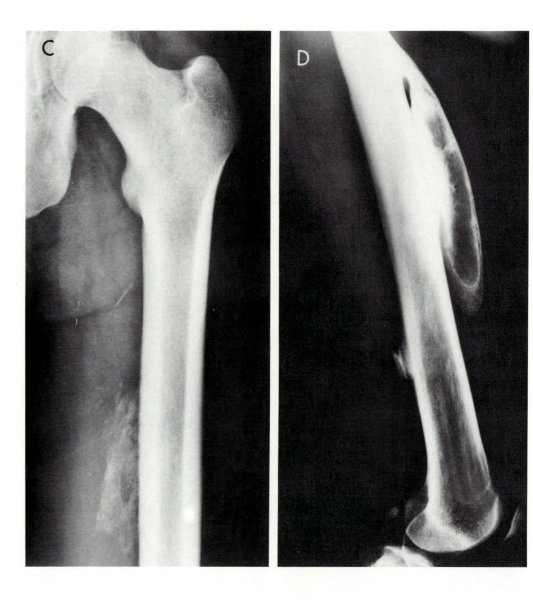

Myositis Ossificans

REMEDY Oral steroids (if acute), ice, range of motion, and quadriceps strengthening exercises. No heat.

Greater Trochanteric Calcific Bursitis

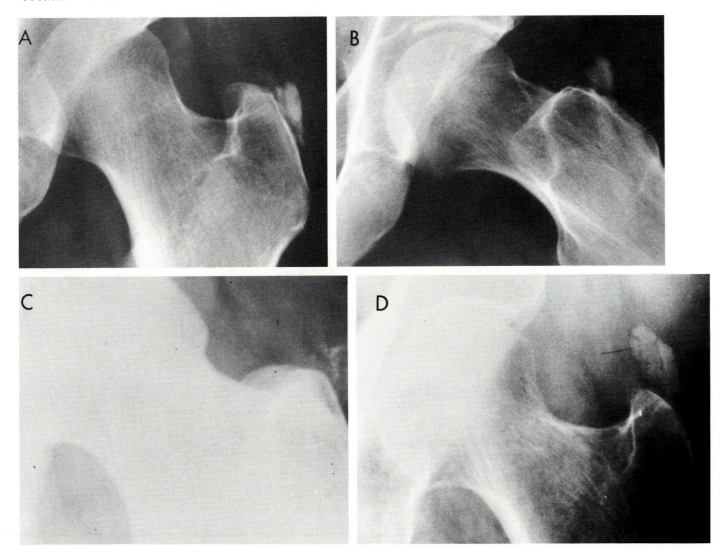

FIG 5–9.
A, B (both same patient), **C, D,** Three examples
of amorphous calcific deposits lateral (**A, B, C**)
and superior (**D**) to the greater trochanter.

Greater Trochanteric Calcific Bursitis

REMEDY Steroid injection. If unresponsive to conservative therapy, surgical excision is recommended.

CHAPTER 6

The Groin

PUBIS

Stress Fracture—Typical

FIG 6–1.
A,B (both same patient), An augmented area of isotope uptake at the right ischial pubic junction.

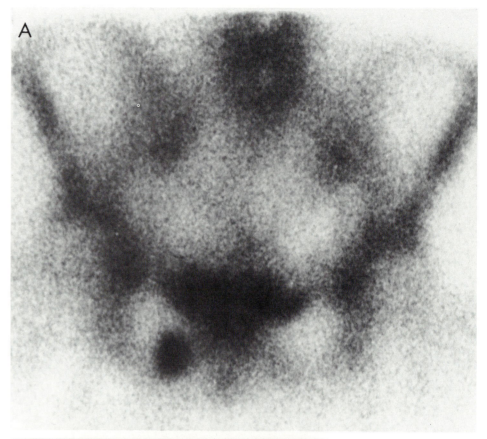

B, A radiograph obtained 10 days later, confirms a stress fracture (*arrowhead*).

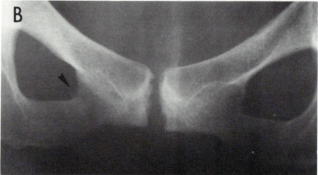

Stress Fracture—Typical

REMEDY   Rest and activity limitation.

Stress Fracture—Nonunion

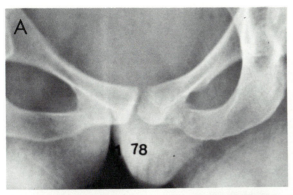

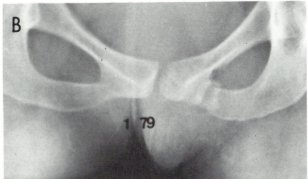

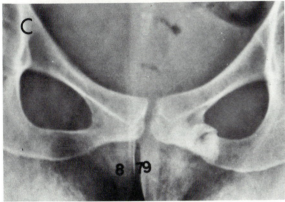

FIG 6–2.
A–C (all same patient), Initial presentation demonstrates a nondisplaced healing stress fracture at the left ischial pubic junction. Two months later (**B**) there is sclerosis bordering the fracture margins and callous formation. The patient continued to run and 7 months later (**C**) there is marked sclerosis bordering the fracture margin representing a nonunion. *(Continued.)*

Stress Fracture—Nonunion (cont.)

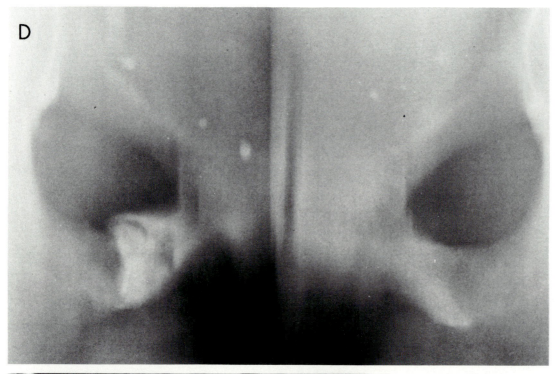

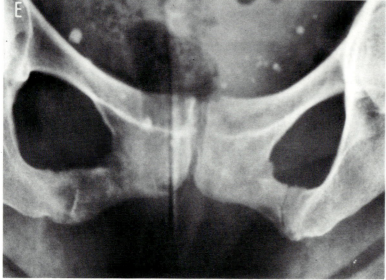

FIG 6–2 (cont.).
D,E (both same patient), Tomogram performed at time of initial x-rays demonstrated nonunion of a fracture of the right pubis at the junction of the ischial pubic junction. Following rest, the patient resumed running and developed pain on the left after a marathon. **E,** Re-x-ray at that time demonstrated the nonunion on the right has healed but there is a new fracture on the left. (Permission for **A–E** granted courtesy of Pavlov H, Nelson T, Warren RF, et al: Stress fractures of the pubic ramus. *J Bone Joint Surg* 1982; 64A:1020.)

Stress Fracture—Nonunion

REMEDY   Rest and activity limitation.

PUBIC SYMPHYSIS

Degenerative Changes and Osteolysis Secondary to Microtrauma

FIG 6–3.
A, Irregularity and cortical loss of the left pubic bone with widening of the symphysis.

B, Irregularity and cortical loss, bilaterally. *(Continued.)*

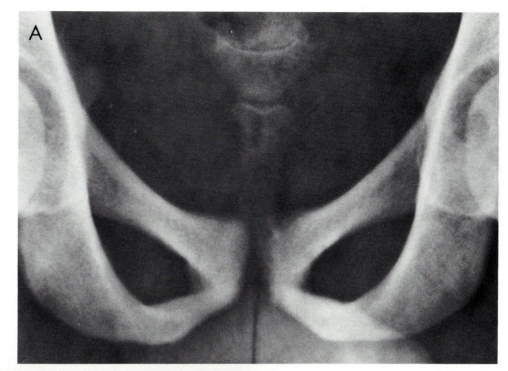

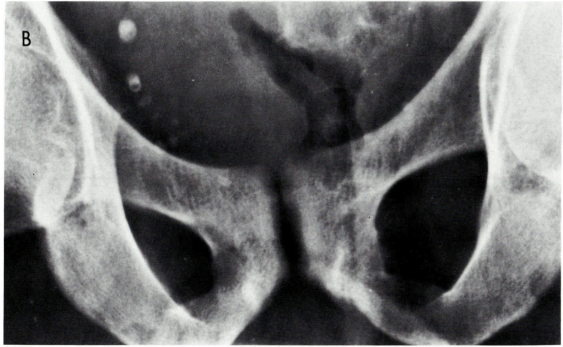

**Degenerative Changes and Osteolysis
Secondary to Microtrauma (cont.)**

FIG 6–3 (cont.).
C, Hypertrophy on the right with
sclerosis inferiorly and cortical irregularity. The inferior portion of the symphysis is widened.

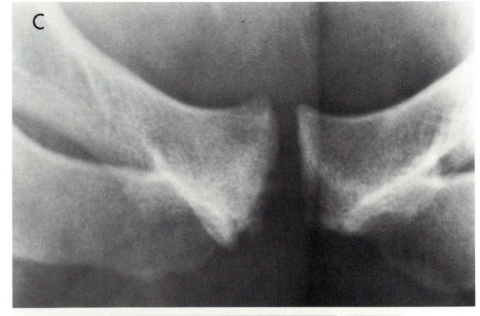

D, Posteroanterior (PA) view demonstrates hypertrophy and sclerosis on
the left with cortical irregularity. The
symphysis is widened. *(Continued.)*

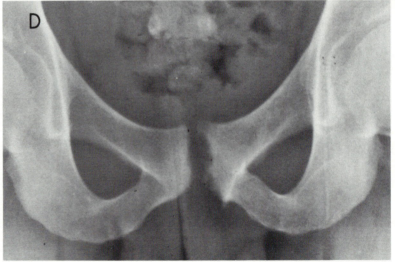

FIG 6–3 (cont.).
E, Marked sclerosis and hypertrophy on the right. The cortex is intact. Symphysis is narrowed.

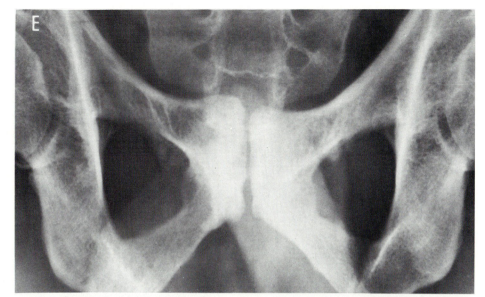

F, Cortical loss bilaterally with large erosions involving the entire left pubis that extends into the inferior pubic ramus. The entire symphysis is widened.

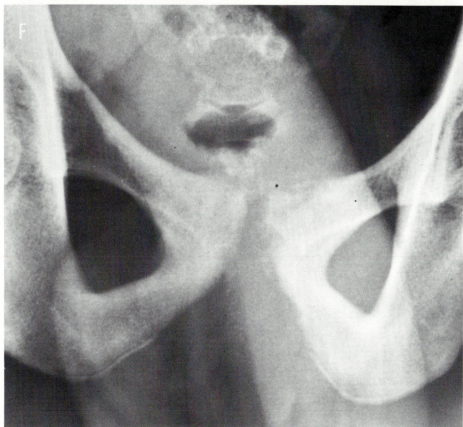

Degenerative Changes and Osteolysis Secondary to Microtrauma

REMEDY   Rest, oral anti-inflammatory drugs, and stretching exercises.

Gracilis Syndrome

"Gracilis syndrome" is a fatigue fracture of traumatic etiology involving bony origin of gracilis muscle at the pubis symphysis. (Ref: Wiley JJ: Traumatic osteitis pubis: The gracilis syndrome. *Am J Sports Med* 1983; 2:360.)

FIG 6–4.
A,B (both same patient), There is an old nondisplaced avulsion fragment at the inferior aspect, left symphysis. The cortex is intact and the symphysis width is maintained.

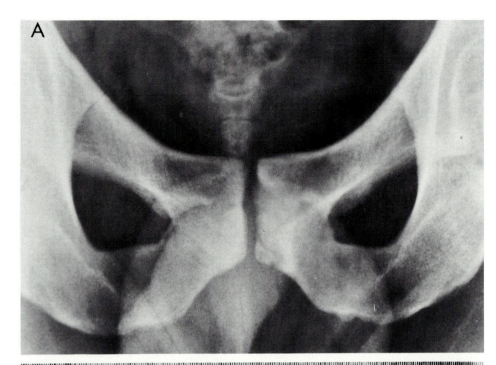

B, On radionuclide bone scan, there is corresponding augmented uptake. *(Continued.)*

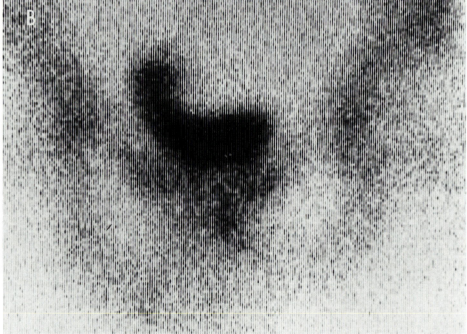

FIG 6–4 (cont.).
C, D, Two examples of gracilis syndrome: there is irregularity of the right pubic cortex with hypertrophy and a well-corticated avulsion fragment inferiorly and spur superiorly.

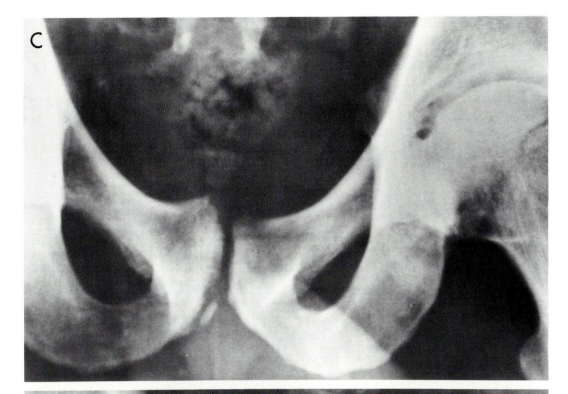

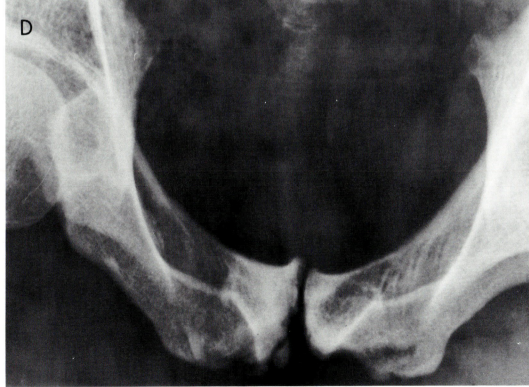

Gracilis Syndrome

REMEDY   Rest, oral anti-inflammatory drugs, and stretching exercises. If conservative treatment is unsuccessful, excision of fragment may be warranted.

Abdominal Rectus Avulsion

FIG 6–5.
Hypertrophy of the right pubic bone with an old avulsion fragment superiorly.

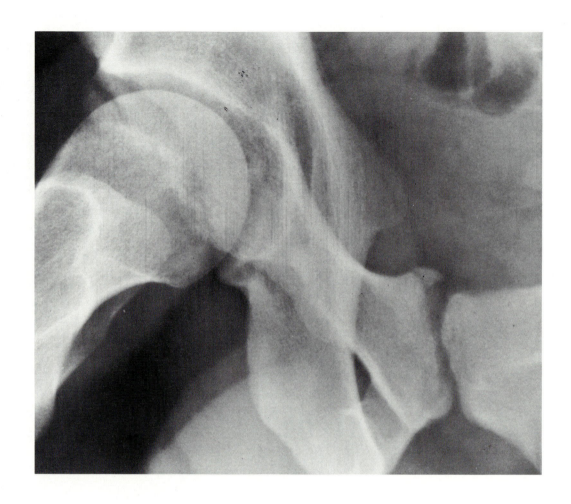

Abdominal Rectus Avulsion

REMEDY   Rest, oral anti-inflammatory drugs, and stretching exercises.

ISCHIUM

Avulsion Injury

Avulsion is secondary to the origin of hamstrings and results from a powerful unbalanced contraction.

FIG 6–6.
A, Bilateral avulsion injuries of the ischia.

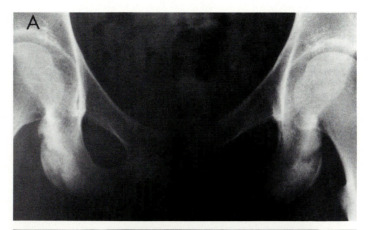

B, Separation of the lateral aspect of the right ischial apophysis *(arrow). (Continued.)*

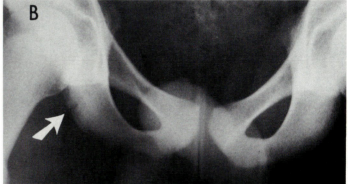

Avulsion Injury (cont.)

FIG 6–6 (cont.).
C, D, E, The avulsion fragment can be widely separated from the bone of origin. *(Continued.)*

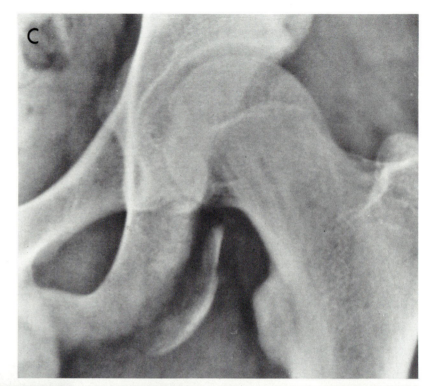

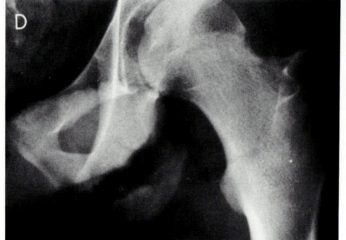

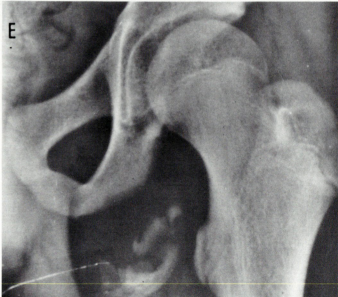

FIG 6–6 (cont.).
F, G (two examples), Healing avulsion fractures of the lateral portion of the left ischial apophysis with abundant calcification.

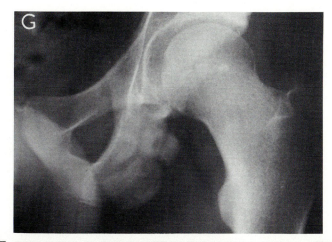

H, A healing avulsion fracture of the ischium producing a mottled appearance with areas of increased density and lucency that simulated a bone tumor.

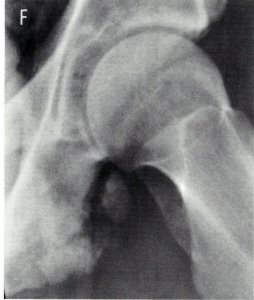

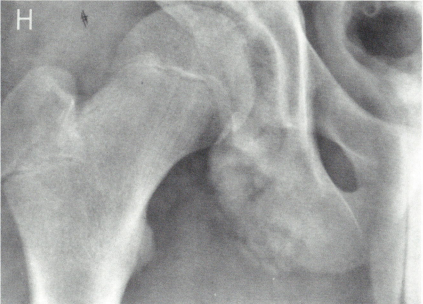

Avulsion Injury

REMEDY   *Initial treatment:* rest, anti-inflammatory drugs, ice, and crutches. If painful *fibrous union* of the avulsed fragment occurs that is unresponsive to conservative management, excision of fragment may be indicated.

ILIUM

Avulsion Injury

Avulsion injuries of the ilium occur at three
sites, the anterior inferior iliac spine and the anterior superior iliac spine, and the iliac cyst apo-
physes.

Anterior Inferior Iliac Spine

Avulsion of the anterior inferior iliac spine is secondary to the reflected head of the rectus fe-
moris origin.

FIG 6–7.
A, B (two examples), Crescent fragment at the
anterior inferior iliac spine and the superolateral
corner of the acetabulum. *(Continued.)*

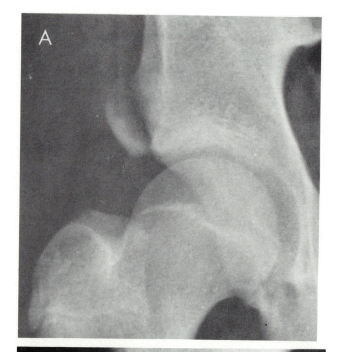

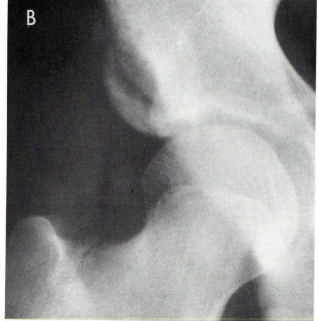

FIG 6–7 (cont.).
C, Healing fracture with amorphous new bone formation in the region of the avulsed fragment at the superior corner of the acetabulum and anterior inferior iliac spine.

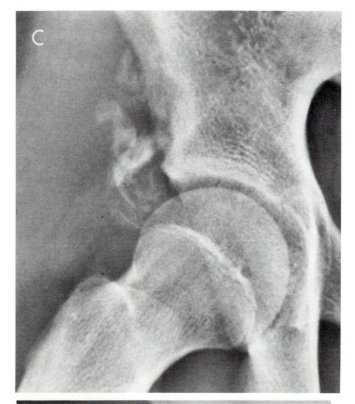

D, Healing avulsion injury with heterotopic ossification superior to the femur. *(Continued.)*

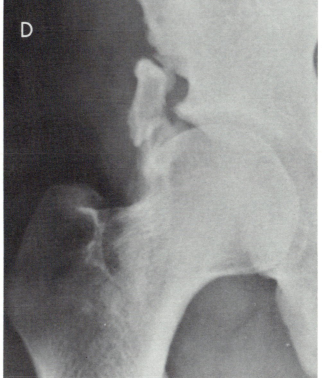

Avulsion Injury (cont.)

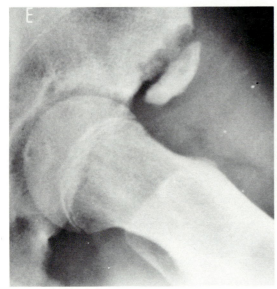

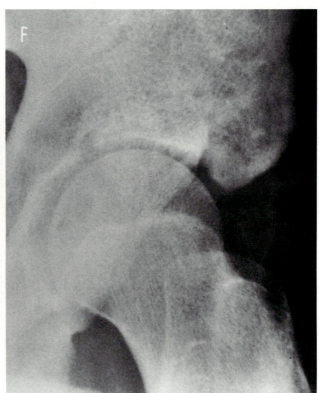

FIG 6–7 (cont.).
E,F (both same patient), Acute avulsion injury.

F, Eventually the fracture healed as a large prominent exostosis. The post-traumatic exostosis typically points toward the joint.

Avulsion Injury—Anterior Inferior Iliac Spine

REMEDY   Rest, ice, and crutches.

Anterior Superior Iliac Spine

Avulsion injuries of the anterior superior iliac spine is secondary to the sartorius and tensor fascia lata origin.

FIG 6–8.
Lateral aspect of anterior superior iliac spine apophysis is displaced. Avulsed fragment can be overlooked if entire ilium is not included in roentgenogram.

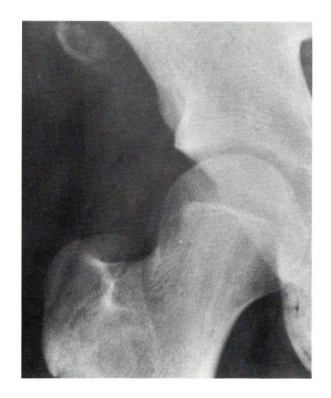

Avulsion Injury—Anterior Superior Iliac Spine

REMEDY   Rest, ice, and crutches. If painful nonunion, excise fragment.

CHAPTER 7

The Spine

CONGENITAL ANOMALIES

Spina Bifida Occulta

FIG 7–1.
Failure of fusion of the posterior neural elements of S1 *(arrow)*, usually of no clinical significance.

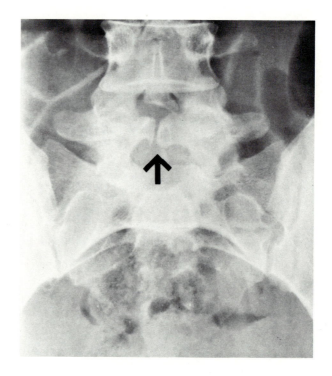

Spina Bifida Occulta

REMEDY None.

Transitional Vertebrae

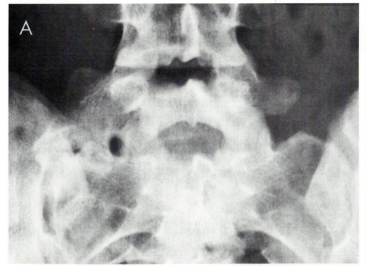

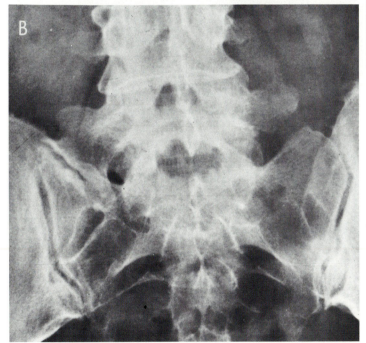

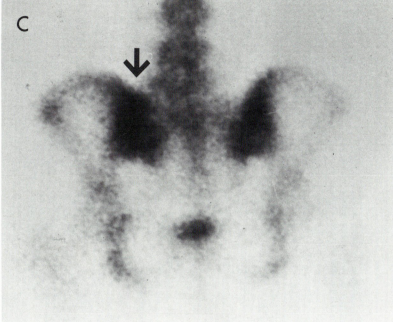

FIG 7–2.
A,C (all same patient), Right transverse process of L5 is broad and attempts articulation to the sacral alae.
B, Coned frontal view of L5–S1 better demonstrates the attempted articulation site between the right transverse process of L5 and the sacrum. The sclerosis bordering the articulation site represents degenerative arthritis secondary to abnormal motion or a pseudoarthrosis.
C, A radionuclide bone scan demonstrates marked augmented isotope uptake *(arrow)* corresponding to the site of pseudoarthrosis.

Transitional Vertebrae

REMEDY   Bed board, Williams' flexion exercises, and activity limitation when symptomatic.

OVERUSE CONDITIONS

Spondylolysis

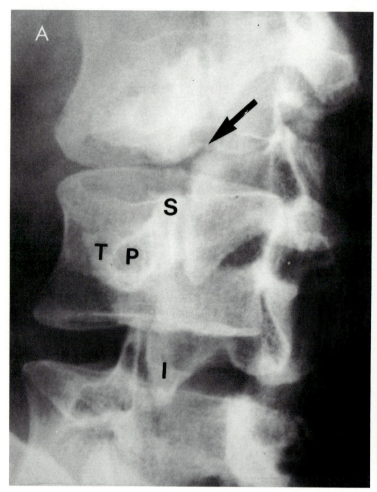

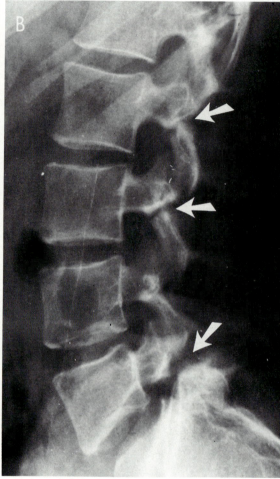

FIG 7–3.
A, A right posterior oblique of the upper lumbar spine demonstrates a spondylolysis of L2 with sclerosis bordering the defect in the pars intra-articularis *(arrow)* representative of a spondylolysis and a nonunion. On this view, the following structures form a "scotty dog" of which the "neck" is the pars intra-articularis; the "ear" is the superior articular facet *(S);* the "eye" is the pedicle *(P);* the "nose" is the transverse process *(T)* and the "front paw" is the inferior articular facet *(I).*

B, Spondylolysis of L2, L3, and L5 *(arrows)* a mild spondylolisthesis of L5–S1 is present. *(Continued.)*

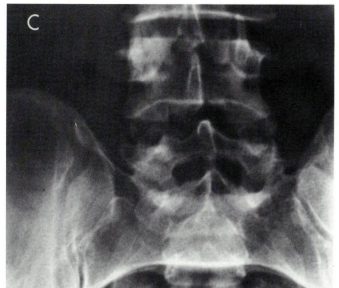

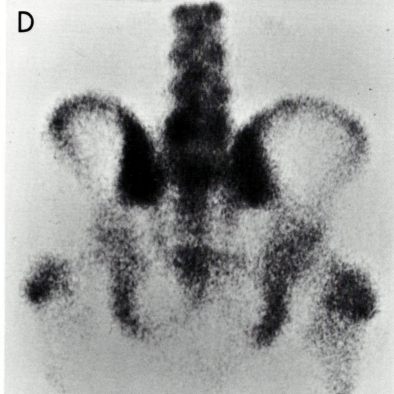

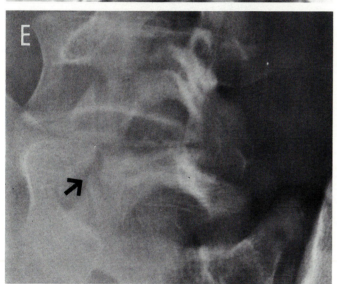

FIG 7–3 (cont.).
C–E (all same patient), The right pedicle of L4 is "white."
D, On a radionuclide bone scan, there is corresponding augmented isotope uptake.
E, A right posterior oblique view demonstrates a spondylolysis of L4 *(arrow). (Continued.)*

Spondylolysis (cont.)

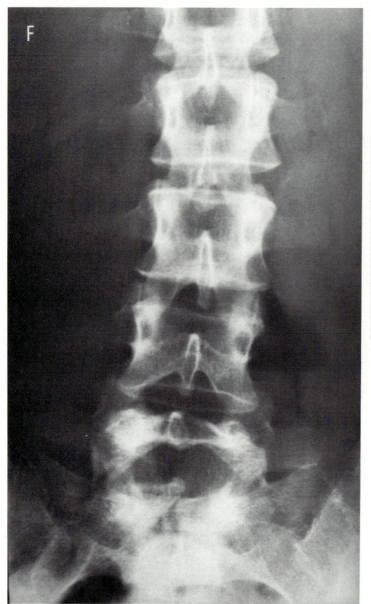

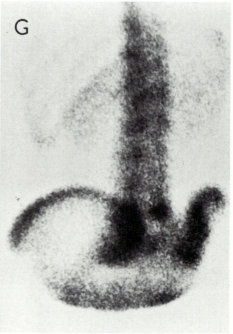

FIG 7–3 (cont.).
F–H (all same patient), There is a slight scoliotic curve, convex to the left. The right L5 pedicle is "white." Incidentally there is a spina bifida occulta of S1.

G, A posterior radionuclide bone scan view demonstrates augmented isotope uptake in the right pedicle of L5. (*Continued.*)

FIG 7–3 (cont.).

H, A left posterior oblique view demonstrates a nondisplaced spondylolysis of the pars interarticularis *(arrows)* on the left. Note the "white" pedicle on the right. Note: the main differential of a "white" pedicle is between an osteoid osteoma or a unilateral spondylolysis. Biopsy of a "white" pedicle is contraindicated because it may be due to a contralateral spondylolysis and biopsy would remove all stability at that level.

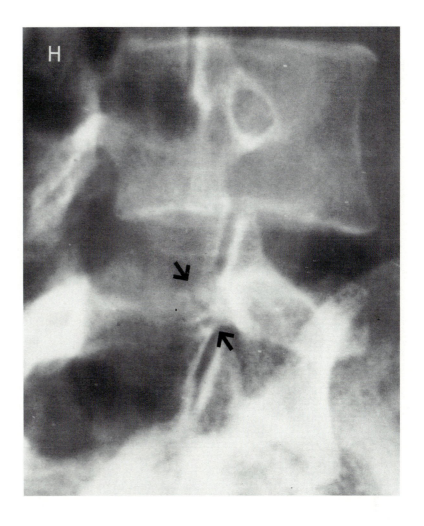

Spondylolysis

REMEDY

Spondylolysis: Patients with spondylolysis can be divided into two groups: (1) preroentgenographic, those with normal roentgenograms and abnormal bone scans; and (2) roentgenographic, those with x-ray evidence of a stress fracture involving the pars. Treatment of both includes limitation of activities, use of a Boston brace, use of a bedboard, Williams flexion exercises, and hamstring stretching, and avoidance of hyperextension activities. Treatment, as outlined, can arrest the preroentgenographic process. Once there is radiographic evidence of stress fracture involving the pars, healing per se does not occur. Treatment will result in the relief of symptoms; however, it will not reverse established roentgenographic findings. Extension of the lumbar spine must be avoided.

Spondylolisthesis should be closely followed for signs of progression, although it is rare for a stress spondylolysis in an athlete to progress to spondylolisthesis.

Intervertebral Disc Disease

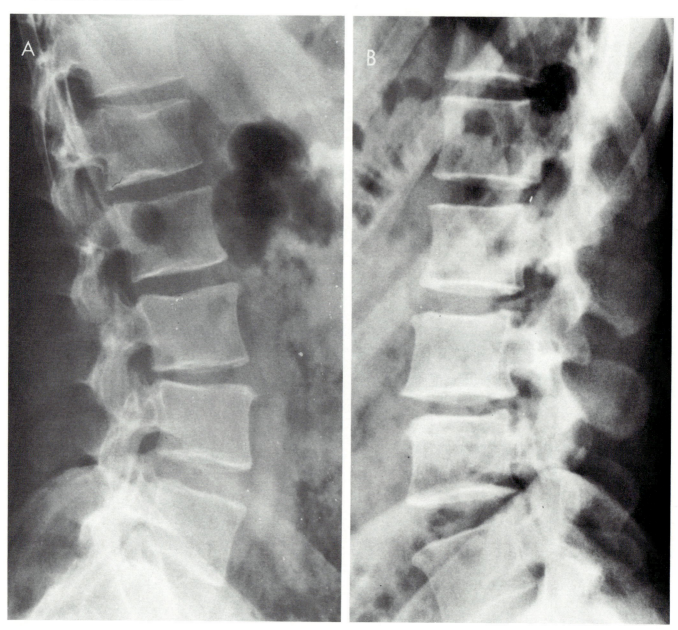

FIG 7–4.
A, Normally, the intervertebral disc spaces gradually enlarge from L1–2 through L4–5 and the L5–S1 intervertebral disc space height is variable. The earliest roentgen demonstration of disc disease is intervertebral disc space narrowing, as seen at L3–4.

B, Radiographic changes of advanced disc disease are increased intervertebral disc space narrowing, sclerosis of the end plates, and hypertrophic spurs as seen between L3–4. *(Continued.)*

FIG 7–4 (cont.).
C, Myelographic demonstration of a bulging disc is present at L3–4 and L4–5. Note the plain film findings of disc space narrowing, discogenic sclerosis (sclerosis bordering the end plates), and proliferative spurs. *(Continued.)*

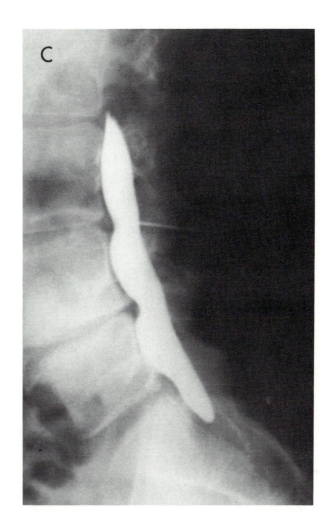

Intervertebral Disc Disease (cont.)

FIG 7–4 (cont.).
D,E (both same patient), Intervertebral disc space narrowing is present at L4–5 on the routine lateral view. *(Continued.)*

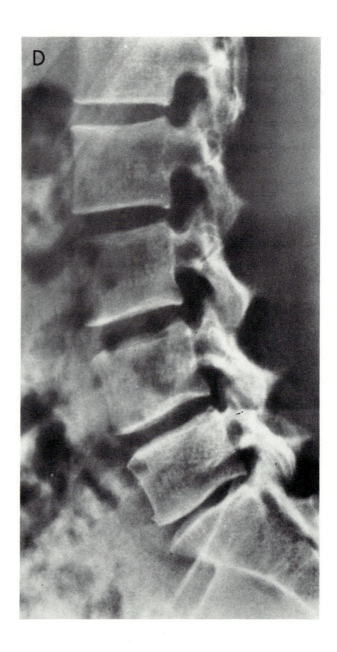

FIG 7–4 (cont.).
E, Discogram demonstrates contrast posterior to the intervertebral disc space at L4–L5 indicating a herniated nucleus pulposus. The L5–S1 disc is degenerated.

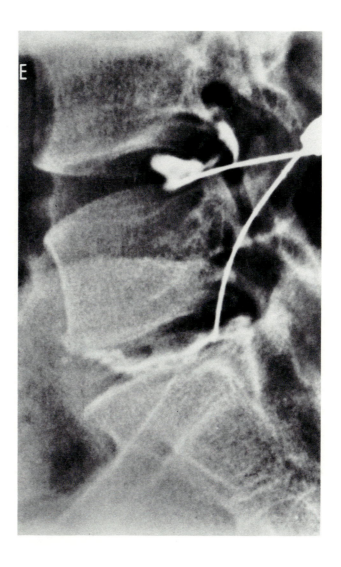

Intervertebral Disc Disease

REMEDY Rest, bed board, muscle relaxants, and analgesics in the acute phase. Williams' flexion exercises, activity modification, and proper lifting techniques with resolution of symptoms. If unresponsive to conservative management, surgery may be indicated.

Suggested Readings

FOOT

General

1. Brody DM: Running injuries. *Clin Symp* 1980; 32(4); 1–36.
2. Torg JS: Sports medicine in the athlete, in Shenker R (ed): *Topics in Adolescent Medicine.* New York, Stratton Intercontinental Medical Book Corp, 1978.

Sesamoids

3. Feldman F, Pochaczevsky R, Hecht H: The case of the wandering sesamoid and other sesamoids afflictions. *Radiology* 1970; 96:275–283.
4. Kidner FC: The prehallux (accessory scaphoid) in its relation to flat-foot. Read at the Joint Meeting of the British and American Orthopaedic Association, London, July 6, 1929.
5. Scranton PE Jr: Pathologic anatomic variations in the sesamoids. *Foot Ankle* 1981; 1(6):321–326.
6. Van Hal ME, Keene JS, Lange TA, et al: Stress fractures of the great toe sesamoids. *Am J Sports Med* 1982; 10(2):122–128.

Metatarsals

7. Kavanaugh JH, Brower TD, Mann RV: The Jones fracture revisited. *J Bone Joint Surg* 1978; 60A:776–782.
8. King JW, Tullos H, Stanley R, et al: Lesions of the feet in athletes. *Southern Med J* 1971; 64:45–48.
9. Micheli LJ, Sohn RS, Solomon R: Stress fractures of the second metatarsal involving Lisfranc's joint in ballet dancers. *J Bone Joint Surg* 1985; 67A:1372–1375.
10. Torg JS, Balduini FC, Zelko RR, et al: Fractures of the base of the fifth metatarsal distal to the tuberosity. *J Bone Joint Surg* 1984; 66A:209–214.

Navicular

11. Devas MB: Compression stress fractures in man and the greyhound. *J Bone Joint Surg* 1961; 43B:540–551.
12. Georgen TG, Venn-Watson EA, Rossman DJ, et al: Tarsal navicular stress fractures in runners. *AJR* 1981; 136:201–203.
13. Main BJ, Jowett RL: Injuries of the midtarsal joint. *J Bone Joint Surg* 1975; 57B:89–97.
14. Pavlov H, Torg JS, Freiberger RH: Tarsal navicular stress fractures: Radiographic evaluation. *Radiology* 1983; 148:641–645.
15. Torg JS, Pavlov H, Cooley LH, et al: Stress fractures of the tarsal navicular. A retrospective review of twenty-one cases. *J Bone Joint Surg* 1982; 63A:700–712.
16. Towne LC, Blazina ME, Cozen LN: Fatigue fracture of the tarsal navicular. *J Bone Joint Surg* 1970; 52A:376–378.
17. Zwelling L, Gunther SF, Hockstein E: Removal of os supranaviculare from a runner's painful foot: A case report. *Am J Sports Med* 1978; 6:1–3.

Talus

18. Fabrikant JM, Hlavac HF: Fracture of the posterior process of the talus in runners. A case report. *J Am Podiatry Assoc* 1979; 69:329–332.

Calcaneus

19. Degan TJ, Morrey BF, Braun DP: Surgical excision for anterior process fractures of the calcaneus. *J Bone Joint Surg* 1982; 64A:519–524.
20. Goldman AB, Pavlov H, Schneider R: Radionuclide bone scanning in subtalar coalitions: Differential considerations. *AJR* 1982; 138:427–432.
21. Norfray JF, Rogers LF, Adamo GP, et al: Common calcaneal avulsion fracture. *AJR* 1980; 134:119–123.
22. Renfrew DL, El-Khoury GY: Anterior process fractures of the calcaneus. *Skeletal Radiol* 1985; 14:121–125.

Posterior Hindfoot

23. Haglund P: Beitrag zur Klinik der Achillessehne. *Z Orthop Chir* 1928; 49:49.

24. Heneghan MA, Pavlov H: The Haglund painful heel syndrome. Experimental investigation of cause and therapeutic implications. *Clin Orthop* 1984; 187:228–234.

25. Heneghan MA, Wallace T: Heel pain due to retrocalcaneal bursitis: Radiographic diagnosis (with an historical footnote on Sever's disease). *Pediatr Radiol* 1985; 15:119–122.

26. Pavlov H, Heneghan MA, Hersh A, et al: The Haglund syndrome: Initial and differential diagnosis. *Radiology* 1982; 144:83.

27. Nidecker AC, Hochstetter A, Fredenhagen H: Accessory muscles of the lower calf. *Radiology* 1984; 151:47–48.

ANKLE

28. Goldman AB, Katz MC, Freiberger RH: Post-traumatic adhesive capsulitis of the ankle: Arthrographic diagnosis. *AJR* 1976; 127:585–588.

29. Pavlov H: Ankle and subtalar arthrography. *Clin Sports Med* 1982; 1(1):47–69.

30. Percy EC, Hill RO, Callaghan JE: The "sprained" ankle. *J Trauma* 1969; 9(12):972–986.

31. Torg JS: Athletic footwear and orthotic appliances. In Ankle and Foot Problems in the Athlete. *Clin Sports Med* 1982; 1:157–175.

LEG

32. Blair WF, Hanley SR: Stress fracture of the proximal fibula. *Am J Sports Med* 1980; 8(3):212–213.

33. Daffner RH: Stress fractures: Current concepts. *Skeletal Radiol* 1978; 2:221–229.

34. Daffner RH, Martinez S, Gehweiler JA, et al: Stress fractures of the proximal tibia in runners. *Radiology* 1982; 142:63–65.

35. Devas MB: Stress fractures of the tibia in athletes or "shin soreness." *J Bone Joint Surg* 1958; 40B:227–239.

36. Geslien GE, Thrall JH, Espinosa JL, et al: Early detection of stress fractures using 99m Tc-Polyphosphate. *Radiology* 1976; 121:683–687.

37. Holder LE, Michael RH: The specific scintigraphic pattern of "shin splints in the lower leg." (Concise communication.) *J Nucl Med* 1984; 25:865–869.

38. Marcia M, Brennan RE, Edeikan J: Computed tomography of stress fractures. *Skeletal Radiol* 1982; 8:193–195.

39. Orava S, Puranen J, Ala-Ketola L: Stress fractures caused by physical exercise. *Acta Orthop Scand* 1978; 49:19–27.

40. Roub LW, Gumerman LW, Hanley EN, et al: Bone stress: A radionuclide imaging perspective. *Radiology* 1979; 132:431–438.

41. Wilcox JR, Moniot A, Green JP: Bone scanning in the evaluation of exercise-related stress injuries. *Radiology* 1977; 123:699–703.

42. Wilson ES, Katz FN: Stress fractures. An analysis of 250 consecutive cases. *Radiology* 1969; 92:481–486.

THE KNEE

General

43. Smillie IS: *Injuries of the Knee Joint* ed 4. New York, Churchill Livingstone, 1970.

Patella

44. Goodfellow J, Hungerford DS, Woods C: Patellofemoral joint mechanics and pathology. II. Chondromalacia patella. *J Bone Joint Surg* 1976; 53B:291.

45. Hensal F, Nelson T, Pavlov H, et al: Bilateral patellar fractures from indirect trauma. A case report. *Clin Orthop* 1983; 178:207.

46. Insall J, Falvo KA, Wise DW: Chondromalacia patella. *J Bone Joint Surg* 1976; 58A:1.

47. Merchant AC, Mercer RL, Jacobsen RH, et al: Roentgenographic analysis of patello-femoral congruence. *J Bone Joint Surg* 1974; 56A: 1391.

Ligaments/Tendons

48. Hughston JC, Andrews JR, Cross MJ: Classification of knee ligament instabilities. I. The medical compartment and cruciate ligaments. *J Bone Joint Surg* 1976; 58A:159.

49. Hughston JC, Andrews JR, Cross MJ: Classification of knee ligament instabilities. III. The lateral compartment. *J Bone Joint Surg* 1976; 58A:173.

50. Pavlov H, Torg JS: Arthrographic evaluation of the knee ligaments. *Contemporary Orthopaedics* 1979; 1(1); 22–26.

51. Nance EP Jr, Kaye JJ: Injuries of the quadriceps mechanism. *Radiology* 1982; 142:301.

52. Woods WG, Rufus SF Jr, Tullos HS: Lateral capsular sign: X-ray clue to a significant knee instability. *Am J Sports Med* 1979; 7(1):27.

Osteochondral Fractures/Osteochondritis Dissecans

53. Cayea PD, Pavlov H, Sherman MF, et al: Lucent articular lesion in the lateral femoral condyle: Source of patellar femoral pain in the athletic adolescent. *AJR* 1981; 137:1145.

54. Lipscomb PR Jr, Lipscomb PR Sr, Bryan RS: Osteochondritis dissecans of the knee with loose fragments. *J Bone Joint Surg* 1978; 60A:235.

55. Milgram JW: Osteochondral fractures: Mechanisms of injury and fate of fragments. *AJR* 1978; 130:651.

56. Milgram JW: Radiological and pathological manifestations of osteochondritis dissecans of the distal femur. *Radiology* 1978; 126:305.

57. Dietz GW, Wilcox DM, Montgomery JB: Segond tibial condyle fracture: Lateral capsular ligament avulsion. *Radiology* 1986; 159:467.

FEMUR

Distal Shaft

58. Butler JE, Brown SL, McConnell BG: Subtrochanteric stress fractures in runners. *Am J Sports Med* 1982; 10(4):228.
59. Lombardo SJ, Benson DW: Stress fractures of the femur in runners. *Am J Sports Med* 1982; 10(4):219.
60. Provost RA, Morris JM: Fatigue fracture of the femoral shaft. *J Bone Joint Surg* 1969; 51A:487.
61. Torg JS, Pavlov H, Morris VB: Salter-Harris type III fracture of the medial femoral condyle occurring in the adolescent athlete. *J Bone Joint Surg* 1981; 63A:586.

Hip

62. Skinner HB, Cook SD: Fatigue failure stress of the femoral neck. A case report. *Am J Sports Med* 1982; 10(4):245.

GROIN

Pubis

63. Latshaw RF, Kantner TR, Kalenak A, et al: A pelvic stress fracture in a female jogger. A case report. *Am J Sports Med* 1981; 9(1):54–56.
64. Pavlov H, Nelson TL, Warren RF, et al: Stress fractures of the pubic ramus. A report of twelve cases. *J Bone Joint Surg* 1982; 64A:1020.

Pubic Symphysis

65. Adams RJ, Chandler FA: Osteitis pubis of traumatic etiology. *J Bone Joint Surg* 1953; 35(A) 3:685–695.
66. Cochrane GM: Osteitis pubis in athletes. *Br J Sports Med* 1971; 5:233–235.
67. El-Khoury GY, Wehbe MA, Bonfiglio M, et al: Stress fractures of the femoral neck: A scintigraphic sign for early diagnosis. *Skeletal Radiol* 1981; 6:271.
68. Hanson PG, Angevine M, Juhl JH: Osteitis pubis in sports activities. *The Physician and Sportsmedicine* 1978; 4:111.
69. House AJG: Osteitis pubis in an Olympic road walker. *Proc R Soc Med* 1964; 57:88–90.

70. Klinefelter EW: Osteitis pubis. Review of the literature and report of a case. *AJR* 1950; 63 (3):368.
71. Koch RA, Jackson DW: Pubic symphysitis in runners. A report of two cases. *Am J Sports Med* 1981; 9(1):62.
72. Peirson EL Jr: Osteochondritis of the symphysis pubis. *Surg Gynecol Obstet* 1929; 49:834.
73. Schnute WJ: Osteitis pubis. *Clin Orthop* 1961; 20:187–192.
74. Schneider R, Kaye JJ, Ghelman B: Adductor avulsive injuries near the symphysis pubis. *Radiology* 1976; 120:567.
75. Vazelle F, Rochcongar P, LeJeune JJ, et al: Le syndrome d'algie pubienne du sportif (pubialgie). *J Radiol* 1982; 63:423.
76. Vix VA, Ryu CY: The adult symphysis pubis: Normal and abnormal. *AJR* 1971; 112 (3):517.
77. Wiley JJ: Traumatic osteitis pubis: The gracilis syndrome. *Am J Sports Med* 1983; 11(5):360.

Ischium

78. Fernbach SK, Wilkinson RH: Avulsion injuries of the pelvis and proximal femur. *AJR* 1981; 137:581.
79. Muckle DS: Associated factors in recurrent groin and hamstring injuries. *Br J Sports Med* 1982; 16(1):37.

Ilium

80. Bavendam FA, Nedeleman SH: Some consideration in the roentgenology of fractures and dislocations. *Semin Roentgenol* 1966; 1:407–436.
81. Clancy WG Jr, Foltz AS: Iliac apophysitis and stress fractures in adolescent runners. *Am J Sports Med* 1976; 4(5):214.
82. Godshall RW, Hansen CA: Incomplete avulsion of a portion of the iliac epiphysis. An injury of young athletes. *J Bone Joint Surg* 1973; 55A:1301.
83. Milgram JE: Muscle ruptures and avulsion with particular reference to the lower extremities, in *The American Academy of Orthopaedic Surgeons Instructional Course Lectures*. Ann Arbor, Edwards, 10, 1953; pp 233–243.

THE SPINE

84. Stanish W: Low back pain in middle-aged athletes. *Am J Sports Med* 1979; 7(6):367.
85. Stanitski CL: Low back pain in young athletes. *Physician and Sportsmedicine* 1982; 10(10):77.

Index